Essential Echocardiography

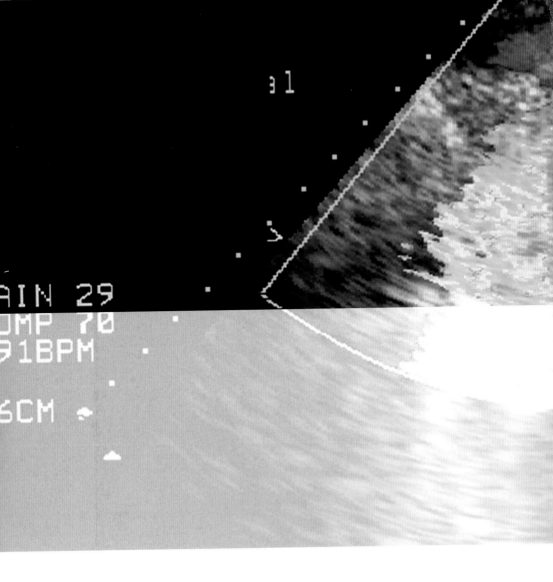

Dedication
For Christine, Grace, Eleanor, Beatrix and my parents

For Elsevier
Content Strategist: Laurence Hunter
Content Development Specialist: Helen Leng
Project Manager: Andrew Riley
Designer/Design Direction: Christian Bilbow
Illustration Manager: Jennifer Rose

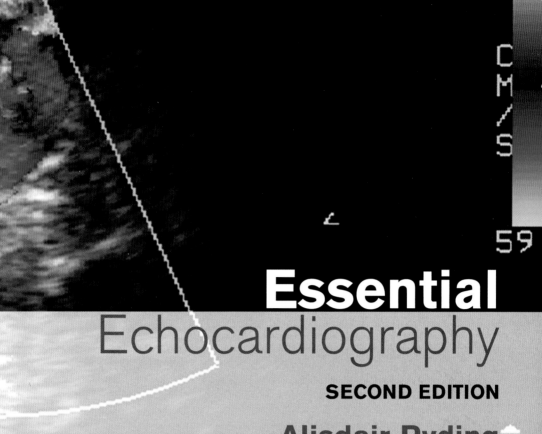

Essential
Echocardiography

SECOND EDITION

Alisdair Ryding

BSc(Med Sci)Hons, MBChB(Hons), MRCP (UK), PhD

Consultant Cardiologist, Norfolk and
Norwich University Hospital; Honorary Consultant
Cardiologist, James Paget University Hospital, Norwich, UK

With a contribution by

James Newton MRCP, MD

Consultant Cardiologist and Clinical Lead for Echocardiography,
Oxford University Hospitals NHS Trust, Oxford, UK

Sayeh Zielke MD, MBA, FRCPC

Cardiac Imaging Fellow, John Radcliffe Hospital, Oxford, UK

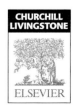

CHURCHILL
LIVINGSTONE

ELSEVIER

Edinburgh   London   New York   Oxford   Philadelphia   St Louis   Sydney   Toronto   2013

CHURCHILL
LIVINGSTONE
ELSEVIER

© 2013 Elsevier Ltd All rights reserved.

No part of this publication may be reproduced or transmitted in any form or by any means, electronic or mechanical, including photocopying, recording, or any information storage and retrieval system, without permission in writing from the publisher. Details on how to seek permission, further information about the publisher's permissions policies and our arrangements with organizations such as the Copyright Clearance Center and the Copyright Licensing Agency, can be found at our website: www.elsevier.com/permissions.

This book and the individual contributions contained in it are protected under copyright by the publisher (other than as may be noted herein).

First edition 2008
Second edition 2013

ISBN 9780702045523

British Library Cataloguing in Publication Data
A catalogue record for this book is available from the British Library

Library of Congress Cataloging in Publication Data
A catalog record for this book is available from the Library of Congress

Notices
Knowledge and best practice in this field are constantly changing. As new research and experience broaden our understanding, changes in research methods, professional practices, or medical treatment may become necessary.

Practitioners and researchers must always rely on their own experience and knowledge in evaluating and using any information, methods, compounds, or experiments described herein. In using such information or methods they should be mindful of their own safety and the safety of others, including parties for whom they have a professional responsibility.

With respect to any drug or pharmaceutical products identified, readers are advised to check the most current information provided (i) on procedures featured or (ii) by the manufacturer of each product to be administered, to verify the recommended dose or formula, the method and duration of administration, and contraindications. It is the responsibility of practitioners, relying on their own experience and knowledge of their patients, to make diagnoses, to determine dosages and the best treatment for each individual patient, and to take all appropriate safety precautions.

To the fullest extent of the law, neither the publisher nor the authors, contributors, or editors assume any liability for any injury and/or damage to persons or property as a matter of products liability, negligence or otherwise, or from any use or operation of any methods, products, instructions, or ideas contained in the material herein.

Printed in China

 ELSEVIER your source for books, journals and multimedia in the health sciences

www.elsevierhealth.com

| Working together to grow libraries in developing countries | The publisher's policy is to use **paper manufactured from sustainable forests** |

www.elsevier.com | www.bookaid.org | www.sabre.org

ELSEVIER   BOOK AID International   Sabre Foundation

Contents

Preface

Echocardiography is an immensely powerful tool, providing a wealth of information about cardiac structure and function. Unlike other imaging modalities this can be achieved painlessly, quickly, safely and at low cost. Echo machines are increasingly portable, and easily used in a wide range of emergency and community settings. No wonder there is huge interest and demand for training in echo by a wide spectrum of healthcare providers.

Echocardiography is a daunting skill to learn, and there are many potential pitfalls for the unsuspecting. How do you get good pictures? How do you distinguish normal and abnormal? Are you making the right measurements and have you made the correct diagnosis? *Essential Echocardiography* was written to provide answers to these questions. It is a practical guide that allows the beginner to become a confident and independent practitioner. The first chapters cover the principles of ultrasound and focus on the practical aspects of performing and optimising an echo. Subsequent chapters systematically look at the various cardiac chambers, valves and extra-cardiac structures in health and disease. There are new chapters on 3D echo and right ventricular pathologies, with more than 200 new images to illustrate state-of-the-art echo.

Particular emphasis has been placed on the knowledge and skills required for image interpretation, reporting and diagnosis: there are over 300 on-line videos to allow you to develop this expertise. Finally I have written 100 on-line interactive self-assessment questions to test your knowledge, understanding and diagnostic skills.

Alisdair Ryding
Norwich, UK

Abbreviations

2D	two-dimensional
3D	three-dimensional
A	transmitral Doppler atrial diastolic wave
a'	annular late diastolic myocardial velocity
A2C	apical two-chamber
A3C	apical three-chamber
A4C	apical four-chamber
A5C	apical five-chamber
AR	atrial regurgitation
ARVD	arrhythmogenic right ventricular dysplasia
ASA	atrial septal aneurysm
ASD	atrial septal defect
ASH	asymmetric septal hypertrophy
AV	atrioventricular/aortic valve
BART	blue away, red towards
bpm	beats per minute
BSA	body surface area
CFM	colour flow mapping
COPD	chronic obstructive pulmonary disease
CRT	cardiac resynchronisation therapy
CT	computed tomography
CW	continuous wave (Doppler)
DSE	dobutamine stress echo
DT	deceleration time
DTI	Doppler tissue imaging
E	transmitral Doppler early diastolic wave
E:A	ratio of E and A wave peak velocities
e'	annular early diastolic myocardial velocity
ECG	electrocardiograph
EF	ejection fraction
EROA	effective regurgitant orifice area
FS	fractional shortening
HCM	hypertrophic cardiomyopathy
HIV	human immunodeficiency virus
HOCM	hypertrophic obstructive cardiomyopathy
IAS	interatrial septum
IE	infective endocarditis
IVC	inferior vena cava
IVS	interventricular septum
IVSd	diastolic interventricular septal thickness
LA	left atrium
LBBB	left bundle branch block
LGC	lateral gain compensation
LV	left ventricle
LVH	left ventricular hypertrophy
LVID	left ventricular internal diameter

LVIDd	end diastolic left ventricular internal diameter
LVIDs	systolic left ventricular internal diameter
LVNC	left ventricular non-compaction
LVOT	left ventricular outflow tract
LVOTO	left ventricular cardiomyopathy obstruction
MAPSE	mitral annular plane systolic excursion
MI	myocardial infarction
MRI	magnetic resonance imaging
MV	mitral valve
MVA	mitral valve area
MVP	mitral valve prolapse
PASP	pulmonary artery systolic pressure
PFO	patent foramen ovale
PISA	proximal isovelocity surface area
PRF	pulse repetition frequency
PSLAX	parasternal long axis
PSSAX	parasternal short axis
PV	pulmonary valve
PW	pulse wave (Doppler)
PWT	posterior wall thickness
PWTd	diastolic posterior wall thickness
RA	right atrium
RMVD	rheumatic mitral valve disease
RV	right ventricle
RVEDP	right ventricular end diastolic pressure
RVOT	right ventricular outflow tract
RVSP	right ventricular systolic pressure
RWMA	regional wall motion abnormality
SAM	systolic anterior motion of the mitral valve
SBP	systolic blood pressure
SLE	systemic lupus erythematosus
SV	stroke volume
TAPSE	tricuspid annular plane systolic excursion
TGC	time gain compensation
THI	tissue harmonic imaging
TOE	transoesophageal echocardiography
TTE	transthoracic echocardiography
VSD	ventricular septal defect
VTI	velocity time integral
WMSI	wall motion score index

Acknowledgements

I am very grateful to my patients, without whom this book would not exist. I am also indebted to my colleagues, particularly:

Second edition
Dr Heeraj Bullock, Mrs Sarah Butcher, Mrs Karen Clifton, Mr Charles Graham, Dr Cairistine Grahame-Clarke, Dr Simon Hansom, Mr Darren Hardy-Shepherd, Miss Emma Lakey, Miss Angela Merrick, Mrs Ruth Mixer, Dr J Newton, Dr Helen Oxenham, Miss Sam Peck, Miss Hayley Reeve, Miss Natalie Sales, Mr Seamus Walker, Mrs Sheila Wood.

First edition
Dr K Asrress, Prof H Becher, Dr S Hussain, Dr P Leeson, Dr A Mitchell, Dr J Newton, Mrs M Priest, Mrs S Ramsay, Dr N Sabharwal, Mrs D Smith, Dr D Sprigings, Mr D Tetley, Dr J Timperley, Dr D Tomlinson, Prof S Westaby, Dr A Wrigley.

I would also like to thank everyone at Elsevier who has helped to make this book a reality, in particular Laurence Hunter and Helen Leng.

Alisdair Ryding
Norwich, UK

What is echocardiography?

Echocardiography is the use of specialised ultrasound equipment to image the structure and function of the heart. It is rather like sonar, in that sound waves are used to locate the position of an object based on the characteristics of the reflected signal, hence the use of the term 'echo'.

It is not necessary to have a detailed knowledge of the physics of ultrasound or the inner workings of an echo machine to be able to use one. However, to obtain the best information it is useful to have a basic idea of the principles and limitations of the technique.

Basic principles

Ultrasound uses very-high-frequency sound waves (typically >1.5 MHz) that are beyond the normal range of hearing (>20 kHz). An echo transducer contains piezoelectric crystals (a ceramic material) that vibrate at high frequency when an electric current is passed through them. They convert electrical energy to ultrasound waves, and ultrasound back to electrical energy. It is therefore able to perform the dual role of emitting and transducing ultrasound.

The basic physical properties of ultrasound waves are the wavelength (λ, distance between equivalent points in adjacent cycles; Fig. 1.1), frequency (f, cycles per second) and velocity (v, direction and speed of travel). The relationship between these factors is described by the equation: $v = f \lambda$.

The velocity of ultrasound depends on the physical properties (density) of the tissue. In soft tissues such as heart muscle, ultrasound travels at 1540 m/s, but it is faster in bone and much slower in air. As ultrasound waves pass through the body, they encounter tissue interfaces of different composition that reflect, scatter or refract the waves, rather like the effects of glass on light (Fig. 1.2). If ultrasound waves are reflected back to the echo probe and detected, a picture of

Figure 1.1

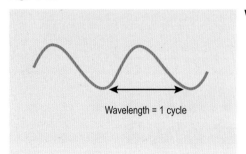

Wavelength.

Wavelength = 1 cycle

Figure 1.2

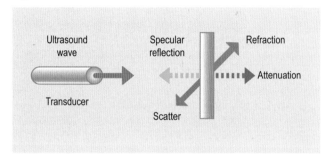

Ultrasound
wave

Transducer

Specular
reflection

Scatter

Refraction

Attenuation

**Ultrasound/tissue
interactions.** Ultrasound
emitted by the transducer (red
arrow) encounters a structure
(rectangle). It may be reflected
directly back (specular reflection:
blue arrow), scattered (green
arrow) or pass through the
tissue and either become
attenuated (purple arrow) or
change course (refraction: dark
blue arrow).

the heart can be built up. This is achieved by working out how long it takes the sound waves to travel to the heart and back: the longer this takes, the further away the structure must be (Fig. 1.3). Therefore an echo machine is continuously processing the raw data received by the transducer to depict what is happening in the heart.

Conveniently, pericardium, endo-/epicardium and valves reflect ultrasound waves strongly (specular reflection), whilst heart muscle causes scattering, and blood causes little reflection at all. These differences in signal intensity allow blood and heart muscle to be easily differentiated on echo.

Echocardiographic modes

Two-dimensional imaging

The most intuitive echo mode is two-dimensional (2D) imaging, sometimes called B-mode, which provides cross-sectional real-time moving images of the heart. There are different ways of achieving this, but most modern echo machines use an array of crystals that are cyclically activated and inactivated in phase. Each cycle effectively produces an arc of ultrasound lines that can be compiled into a 2D image (Fig. 1.4). Repetition of this process hundreds of times per second allows the motion of the heart to be appreciated. The quality of the image is determined

Figure 1.3

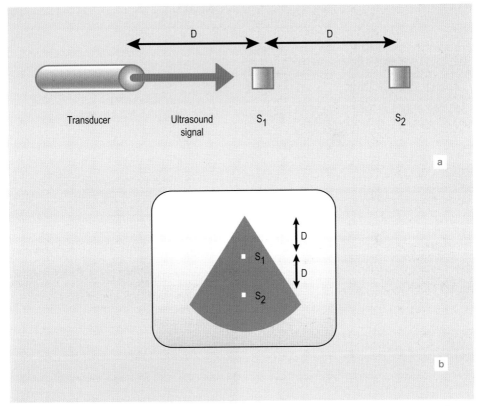

Determination of relative distance. (a) The time elapsing between the emission and receipt of ultrasound signals allows the distance (D) between structures to be calculated. If an ultrasound signal (red arrow) is emitted from the transducer the time taken for this to be reflected back to the transducer by structure S_2 will be twice the time taken for reflection back from structure S_1. **(b)** The visual representation of S_1 and S_2 on the echo screen: the transducer is considered to be at the apex of the triangular sector.

by the number of scan lines (usually over 100 per sector), and the frequency at which they are repeated (frame rate: usually about 100 per second).

Three-dimensional imaging

Real-time three-dimensional imaging is now available and is increasingly used in routine clinical practice. This is discussed in detail in Chapter 21.

M-mode imaging

At one time this was the only available echo mode. It uses a small group of crystals to produce a single narrow beam of ultrasound, which can be analysed to locate the distance of structures from the transducer. 2D images are used to guide placement of the M-mode cursor across the structures of interest. The beam is repeated 1000s of times per second, and each analysis of distance is plotted against time

Figure 1.4

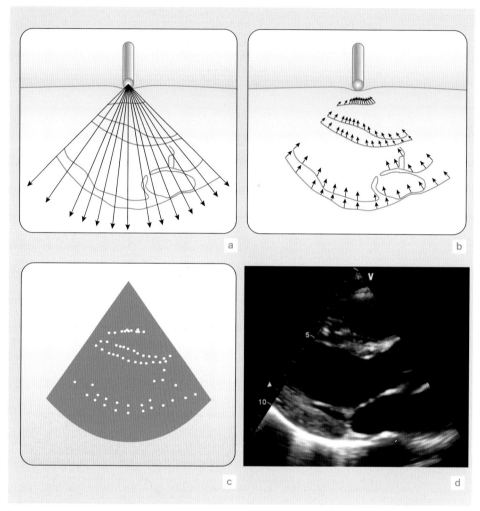

Principle of two-dimensional imaging. (a) Multiple ultrasound beams are emitted, forming an arc of ultrasound that passes through the structures of the chest, including the heart. **(b)** Ultrasound is scattered and reflected at tissue/blood interfaces back towards the transducer. **(c)** The relative positions and timings of each reflected wave allow a two-dimensional picture of the heart to be displayed. Clearly, increasing the number of scan lines will improve the image quality. **(d)** Actual two-dimensional image.

(Fig. 1.5). The advantage of this mode is the very high frame rate, so that the spatial resolution of moving structures is very good, and highly accurate measures of cardiac dimensions can be achieved. The disadvantages are that the images can be difficult to interpret, and reliable measurements require very good technique.

Doppler ultrasound

Doppler ultrasound is a method of detecting the direction and speed of blood flow. Blood cells reflect ultrasound waves like other tissues, but as they are moving, the

Figure 1.5

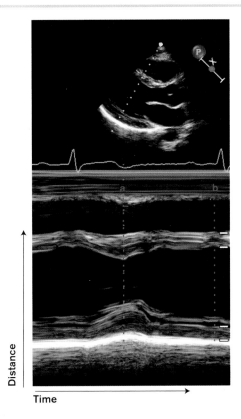

Distance

Time

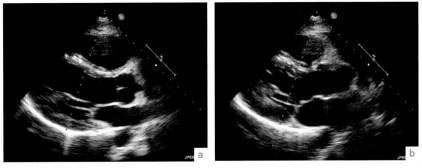

M-mode recordings. M-mode uses a single narrow ultrasound beam to obtain information about the distance of structures from the transducer. The placement of the ultrasound beam (red dotted line) is usually guided by the two-dimensional images. The output is a graphical plot of distance against time. The relationship of diastole and systole to the M-mode picture is indicated by the red lines on the two-dimensional images (**a** and **b**).

frequency of the reflected ultrasound is altered. This distortion is known as the Doppler shift, and is familiar to us in the way an ambulance siren appears to change pitch as it approaches or disappears (Fig. 1.6). Since the frequency of the emitted ultrasound is fixed and predetermined, the change in frequency of the reflected wave tells us the direction and velocity of blood flow: an increase in

Figure 1.6

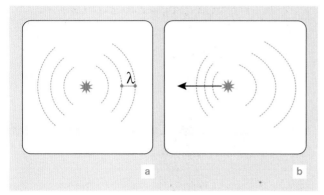

The Doppler principle. (a) A stationary source (star) emits a sound at a certain wavelength, λ (dashed lines). **(b)** If the source moves to the left, the wavelength in that direction shortens, and the frequency increases. Conversely, in the opposite direction there is an apparent increase in wavelength, and drop in frequency.

Figure 1.7

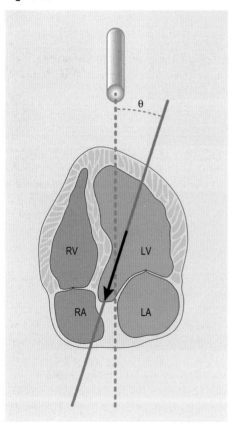

Effect of alignment on Doppler. An apical five-chamber view of the heart is illustrated. The arrow represents blood flow out of the left ventricular outflow tract, travelling at velocity *v*. The dashed line represents the Doppler ultrasound beam, which makes an angle θ with the blood flow. As long as the angle θ remains <20° there is negligible effect on the accuracy of the velocity measurement.

frequency indicates movement towards the transducer, and the greater the shift, the faster the movement. Of course, only the component (vector) of flow that is in line with the ultrasound beam will be detected (Fig. 1.7). If blood is flowing perpendicular to the beam, it cannot be detected. The relationship between the Doppler shift and the speed and direction of blood flow is given in Appendix 2.

Figure 1.8

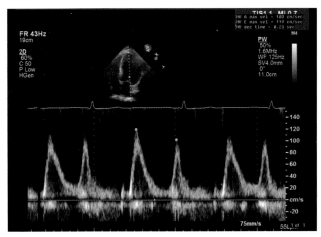

Pulse wave Doppler. Pulse wave Doppler has been used to interrogate blood flow across the mitral valve. Note that blood flow is low-velocity and relatively laminar.

Echo machines can use Doppler information in three ways: pulse wave (PW), continuous wave (CW) and colour flow mapping (CFM). Pulse and CW Doppler are collectively known as spectral Doppler techniques.

Pulse wave Doppler

As the name suggests, PW Doppler uses discrete bursts of ultrasound with gaps in transmission that allow the reflected wave to be received. It is optimised to enable analysis of blood flow at a specific location (represented by the sample volume dot or box on the cursor). This information is displayed graphically as velocity (y-axis) versus time (x-axis), and by convention, blood flow towards the probe is represented above the line (Fig. 1.8).

The fine spatial resolution of PW Doppler is obtained at the expense of velocity resolution, and the detectable velocity range is generally limited to around 1.6 m/s or less. Above this, a phenomenon called *aliasing* occurs, whereby the direction of blood flow appears to be reversed. This is represented graphically by the spectral signal 'wrapping around' to appear on the opposite side of the display (Fig. 1.9). The aliasing velocity depends on the pulse repetition frequency (PRF) used (i.e. number of ultrasound pulses per second), since this determines the maximal detectable Doppler frequency shift, known as the Nyquist limit. The technical reasons for this are complex, but the Nyquist limit is simply equal to half the PRF.

Aliasing occurs when the Doppler frequency shift exceeds the Nyquist limit. The aliasing velocity can be increased to some extent by either using a lower-frequency transducer, or by reducing the image depth to sector size (to increase PRF).

PW Doppler is used to analyse low-velocity blood flow at the mitral valve, in the right and left ventricular outflow tracts and in the pulmonary and hepatic veins. It is also used for quantitative echocardiography. If blood flow is laminar (i.e. uniform velocity), the Doppler spectrum is displayed as a single distinct line (Fig. 1.8). By contrast, turbulent flow comprises many different velocities and directions and this is displayed as a filled-in spectrum.

Figure 1.9

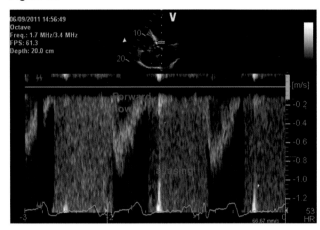

Aliasing. Pulse wave Doppler sampling in the left ventricular outflow tract detects forward flow in systole. The velocity of aortic regurgitation in diastole exceeds the Nyquist limit (1.2 m/s) and the signal 'wraps around' the *y*-axis (aliasing), erroneously indicating forward flow.

Figure 1.10

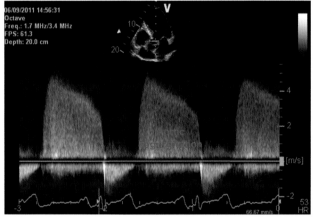

Continuous wave Doppler. Same patient as in Figure 1.9. Continuous wave Doppler has been used to measure the velocity of blood flow across the aortic valve. High-velocity aortic regurgitation is correctly displayed. Note the velocity scale is almost 5 m/s.

Continuous wave Doppler

Continuous emission of ultrasound solves the velocity limitations of PW Doppler by sacrificing spatial resolution, so it is not possible to know exactly where blood flow is localised along the ultrasound beam. For example, CW Doppler cannot distinguish between a gradient across the aortic valve or an obstruction in the left ventricular outflow tract. Careful positioning of the ultrasound cursor on 2D imaging, with guidance from colour flow Doppler, usually allows the CW Doppler data to be interpreted with confidence (Fig. 1.10). This technique is used routinely to measure gradients across stenotic valves.

Colour flow mapping

CFM is basically a pictorial representation of PW Doppler data obtained from a larger area. This is achieved by simultaneously acquiring PW Doppler data from

Figure 1.11

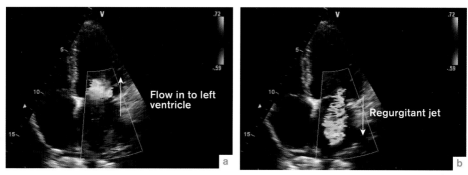

Colour flow mapping (CFM) Doppler. Apical four-chamber views. **(a)** In diastole the majority of blood flows from the left atrium to the left ventricle, towards the probe. This is represented by the red/yellow coloration of the CFM Doppler. **(b)** In systole blood accelerates away from the probe (blue) and exits the left ventricle via the aortic valve (not seen). In this example there is also a jet of mitral regurgitation, which is coloured a mixture of blue, red and yellow due to aliasing caused by the high-velocity turbulent flow.

View **On-line** Images

multiple sample volumes that cover the area of interest. Colours are assigned to represent the direction and velocity of flow, and by convention, blood flowing away from the probe is coded blue, and red towards (BART: blue away, red towards) (Fig. 1.11). Speed of flow is coded according to shades within this scale. It is important to realise that the colour image is simply a computer representation of blood *velocity*, and does not necessarily equate to *volume* of blood flow.

Because this is a PW Doppler technique it is subject to the same velocity limitations, and when aliasing occurs, an inappropriate colour is assigned to the jet of blood flow. This tends to occur at sites of turbulent flow and with valvular regurgitation where velocities can be high (Fig. 1.11b).

CFM is very useful for detecting regurgitant flow at valves, turbulent flow at obstructions, localising shunts and aligning spectral Doppler with blood flow.

Doppler tissue imaging (DTI)

The Doppler techniques described so far are optimised for analysing blood flow, but it is also possible to focus on cardiac tissue movement instead. Unlike blood flow, this is low-velocity, but high-amplitude.

Colour mapping DTI is equivalent to CFM Doppler, in that myocardium is coloured according to its speed and direction of movement (Fig.1.12a and b). A red–blue scale is used with movement towards the transducer coloured red, and blue away (BART). It is important to appreciate that it does not analyse the spatial displacement of myocardium, but the direction and speed. Different tones of red and blue are assigned according to the exact velocity. This technique can be used to look for regional differences in cardiac function.

Spectral DTI analyses the velocity of a small volume of tissue, in much the same way PW Doppler is used to interrogate the velocity of blood flow in a specific sample volume. The sample volume is localised using the 2D/colour DTI image. Data is represented graphically as myocardial velocity versus time. By convention movement towards the transducer is represented above the line (Fig. 1.12c).

Figure 1.12

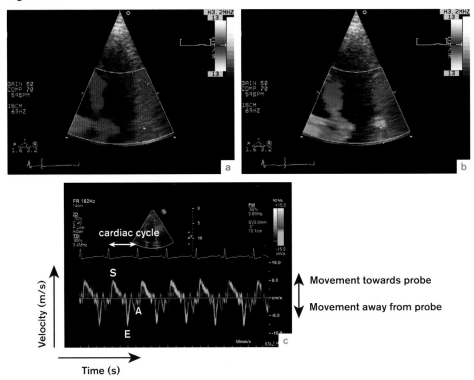

Doppler tissue imaging (DTI). (a and **b)** Tissue Doppler colour mapping. **(c)** Pulse wave spectral tissue Doppler. Colour mapping is overlaid on the two-dimensional image of the myocardium. Red indicates movement towards the probe (systole), and blue away (diastole). Spectral DTI is obtained by placing the sample volume at the desired point. **(c)** An example of pulse wave DTI focused on the lateral mitral annulus is shown. The data is displayed graphically as myocardial velocity versus time. Movement towards the probe is above the line. Note the complex changes in velocity in both systole (S wave) and diastole (E and A waves).

   In clinical practice DTI is specifically used to analyse left ventricular wall motion velocity. During systole, when myocardial contraction occurs there is inward acceleration, followed by deceleration to a standstill as systole ends. In diastole the myocardium relaxes and ventricular filling causes outward acceleration, which again slows and stops until systole resumes. Within this basic description more complex patterns of myocardial acceleration and deceleration occur that provide useful information about systolic and diastolic left ventricular function. This is discussed in more detail in Chapter 5.

Views of the heart

The anatomy of the heart

We all have some idea of the structure of the heart, but you may be surprised at how the heart appears on echo. This is partly because you can only see a two-dimensional cross-section, but also because the structure and orientation of a normal heart are complex. On top of this, you have to get used to the quirks of echocardiographic convention, in which views are almost always displayed with the probe at the top of the screen, so that sometimes everything appears to be upside down. After some practice you will train your eyes to recognise landmarks and orientation will become easy.

It is helpful to think of how the heart is positioned in the chest so that the echocardiographic views are more understandable (Fig. 2.1). The major vessels enter and leave the base of the heart in the centre of the mediastinum, with the apex positioned down to the left, below the nipple. The base is therefore above the apex. If you imagine a sword piercing the chest near the left nipple, and exiting near the right shoulder, this would roughly follow the longitudinal axis of the heart.

The chambers of the heart are oriented such that the right ventricle lies at the front of the chest, and it is wrapped around the left ventricle, in a banana shape. The most posterior structure is the left atrium. Surprisingly the aortic valve and aortic root lie in the centre of everything on most views, and the other valves are clustered around this.

Standard echocardiographic windows

The heart can only be seen from specific points on the chest because ribs and air-filled lung obstruct ultrasound waves. The standard echocardiographic windows include (Fig. 2.2):

Figure 2.1

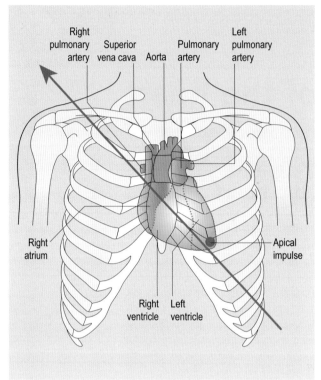

Orientation of the heart in the chest and mediastinum. The longitudinal axis of the heart is roughly from the location of the apex beat to the right shoulder.

Figure 2.2

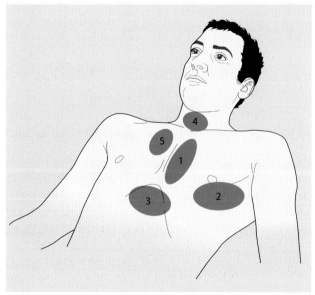

Standard echocardiographic windows. Approximate positions of echo windows are shown in green. Try different rib spaces to obtain the best possible images. 1, Left parasternal; 2, apical; 3, subcostal; 4, suprasternal; 5, right parasternal.

Figure 2.3

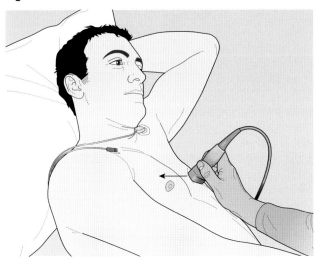

Positioning the patient. For optimal pictures allow the patient to recline at 45°, lying on the left-hand side, with the left arm behind the head. If necessary, try rolling the patient further to the left. The transducer is positioned for the parasternal long axis view, with the marker on the transducer pointing towards the right shoulder of the patient (arrow).

- Left parasternal window
- Apical window
- Subcostal window
- Suprasternal window
- Right parasternal window

These allow the heart to be viewed in most people, but sometimes it is a case of making the most of what information is there.

To obtain the best possible images the patient should recline at 45°, rolled on the left-hand side, with the left arm behind the head, and the right arm by the side (Fig. 2.3). This brings the heart forward, and opens out the rib spaces. Asking the patient to breathe out and hold the breath can improve image quality for parasternal views, by reducing the volume of the lungs and eliminating respiratory movement. A slight breath in can improve apical views.

Positioning yourself and holding the probe

Sit yourself by the patient's right-hand side, so that you are comfortable and stable. Extend your right arm round the patient to reach the echo windows at the front of the chest. Try to keep your spine in a vertical posture because if you have to bend over the patient you will become uncomfortable very quickly!

The transducer should be held loosely like a pen between the thumb and first two fingers (Fig. 2.4). Most probes have a notch or mark that is used for orientation, and start off with this facing upwards. A small amount of ultrasound gel should be applied to the tip of the transducer before holding it gently against the chest in the position you want. It is not necessary to press hard, as this will become uncomfortable for both the patient and yourself. You will rarely get a perfect view first time, but small adjustments in the probe position will often make huge differences in image quality.

Figure 2.4

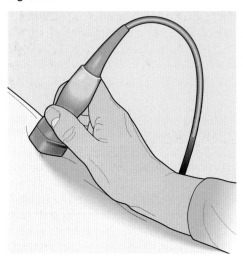

Holding the echo transducer. The transducer should be held like a pen, using the thumb and first and second fingers. Rest the hand and probe gently on the patient's chest. Make small adjustments in position to improve image quality.

Figure 2.5

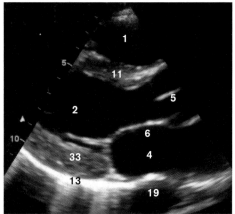

Parasternal long axis view.

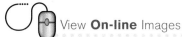 View **On-line** Images

It is also possible to sit and scan from the patient's left-hand side as this can reduce back strain: choose whatever suits you.

Standard views

Parasternal long axis (PSLAX) view

This view is obtained by placing the transducer at the left parasternal edge in the third or fourth intercostal space (Figs 2.2 and 2.3). Try different rib spaces to obtain the best picture. The transducer should be aligned so that the marker is pointing towards the patient's right shoulder.

This view shows many structures (Fig. 2.5), including the mitral and aortic valves, aortic root, left atrium and the base/mid-segments of the left ventricle. The apex of the left ventricle is not usually seen. Ideally the image should be oriented so that the interventricular septum is perpendicular to an M-mode cursor line from the apex of the scan sector. Part of the mid right ventricle is also seen, and further images of the right heart can usually be obtained by angling the beam of the echo probe downwards to see the tricuspid valve from the right atrium (Fig. 2.6a: right ventricular inflow view), or angling upwards to see the pulmonary valve and outflow tract curving round the aortic valve (Fig. 2.6b: right ventricular outflow view).

Parasternal short axis (PSSAX) view

A short axis view of the heart is obtained by rotating the transducer 90° clockwise towards the left shoulder from the PSLAX view (Fig. 2.7). In this view a ring-shaped cross-section of the left ventricle is obtained, with the right ventricle 'stuck' on the side (Fig. 2.8a). Correct orientation for the mid ventricular cut is such that the papillary muscles are seen posteriorly, without the mitral valve leaflets intruding in the picture. If the left ventricle appears oval rather than round, try rotating the probe initially before altering the tilt of the probe.

If the beam is angled downwards (caudally) along the length of the left ventricle it is possible to visualise the left ventricular apex. Scanning with the opposite angulation first reveals the mitral valve in cross-section (Fig. 2.8b): more extreme upward angulation shows the aortic valve in cross-section with the tricuspid valve, right ventricular outflow tract and pulmonary valve curving round the left heart (Fig. 2.8c).

Figure 2.6

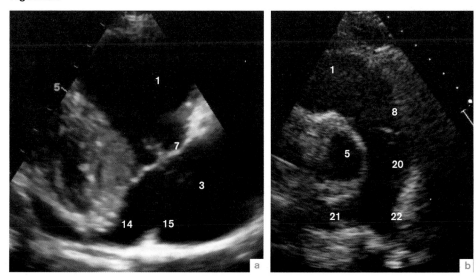

Modified parasternal long axis views.
(a) Downward tilt: right ventricular inflow view. **(b)** Upward tilt: right ventricular outflow view.

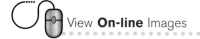

View **On-line** Images

Figure 2.7

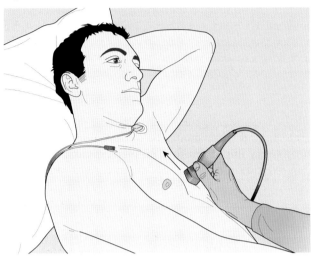

Parasternal short axis view.
The probe is rotated 90°
clockwise from the parasternal
long axis view position so that
the marker now points towards
the patient's left shoulder (arrow).

Figure 2.8

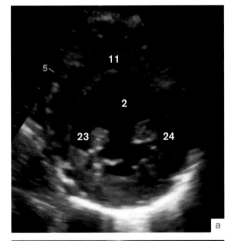

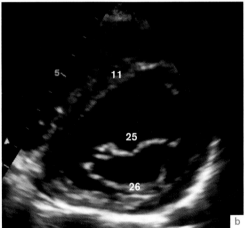

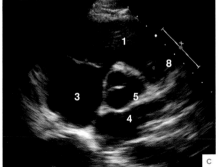

Parasternal short axis views. (a) Mid ventricular
level. **(b)** Mitral valve level. **(c)** Aortic valve level.

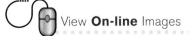

View **On-line** Images

Apical views

The next major view is to look at the heart from the apex, with the transducer marker directed to the patient's left-hand side (Fig. 2.9). The best position is usually a matter of trial and error. Try different rib spaces and locations to optimise the picture orientation and image quality. A common mistake is to hold the probe too high up/central in the chest.

The apical four-chamber (A4C) view shows both ventricles, both atria and the mitral and tricuspid valves (Fig. 2.10a). Ideally the interventricular septum should run down the middle of the screen, and there should be no foreshortening of the left ventricular apex. This view is very important for Doppler examination of the mitral and tricuspid valves, as well as estimation of left and right ventricular function.

The apical five-chamber view (A5C view) incorporates the left ventricular outflow tract (LVOT) as a fifth chamber. It is obtained with slight upward angulation of the echo beam, bringing the LVOT and aortic valve into view (Fig. 2.10b). This view is important for Doppler measurements of the LVOT and aortic valve.

The apical two-chamber view (A2C view) involves rotation of the echo probe from the standard apical four-chamber view, approximately 45° anticlockwise, so that the marker points towards the left shoulder. This shows the anterior and inferior left ventricular walls (Fig. 2.10d).

The apical three-chamber view (A3C) requires further rotation 45° anticlockwise, so that the probe marker is pointing towards the right shoulder. This is very similar to the PSLAX view, but in a different orientation (Fig. 2.10c).

Subcostal views

Subcostal views should be used routinely in all patients. Many of the parasternal and apical views can be replicated from this position, allowing confirmation of

Figure 2.9

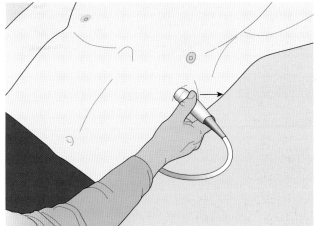

Apical window. The transducer is positioned near the apex of the left ventricle. The exact position varies between people, and you should find the position that gives the best views without 'foreshortening' the left ventricle. The probe marker is directed to the left.

Figure 2.10

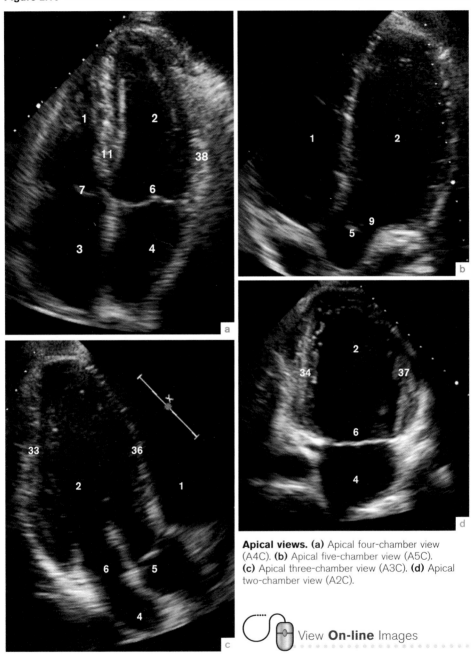

Apical views. (a) Apical four-chamber view (A4C). **(b)** Apical five-chamber view (A5C). **(c)** Apical three-chamber view (A3C). **(d)** Apical two-chamber view (A2C).

View **On-line** Images

previous findings. In immobile patients, particularly those in intensive care, these are frequently the only views obtainable.

With the patient in a semi-recumbent position, and the knees drawn up slightly to relax the abdomen, the probe is placed under the centre of the ribcage (xiphisternum), aiming for the left shoulder with the probe marker pointing towards the patient's left (Fig. 2.11). The best views are often obtained if the patient breathes in and holds the breath.

This view provides an off-axis four-chamber view (Fig. 2.12a). Slight upward tilt can bring the aortic valve/LVOT into view, simulating an A5C view. Rotating the probe 90° anticlockwise provides short axis views of the left and right ventricles (Fig. 2.12b). Further upward angulation of the probe can image the aortic valve in cross-section, together with the right heart structures (Fig. 2.12c).

Swinging the transducer towards the patient's right-hand side allows the inferior vena cava and hepatic veins to be visualised (Fig. 2.12d).

Suprasternal views

This window allows parts of the thoracic aorta to be viewed. The patient should recline at 45°, with the head tilted backwards. The transducer is positioned in the supraclavicular fossa at the base of the neck with the notch towards the left shoulder. In this position the aortic arch and descending aorta are seen (Fig. 2.13), whilst manipulating the transducer towards the right shoulder enables the ascending aorta to be seen (Fig. 2.14a). Use colour flow mapping (CFM) Doppler to demonstrate blood flow in order to help identify the aorta and its branches. Rotating the transducer 45° anticlockwise provides a short axis view, allowing the posterior portion of the left atrium and pulmonary venous inflow to be viewed (Fig. 2.14b). This is known as the crab view, due to the configuration of the left atrium and the four pulmonary veins.

Figure 2.11

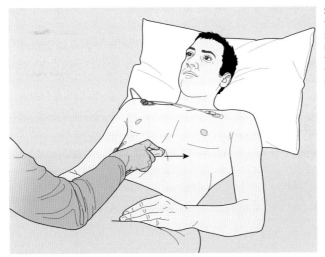

Subcostal views. The transducer is placed under the xiphisternum, where the ribcage meets the sternum, pointing towards the left shoulder. The transducer is oriented towards the patient's left-hand side.

Figure 2.12

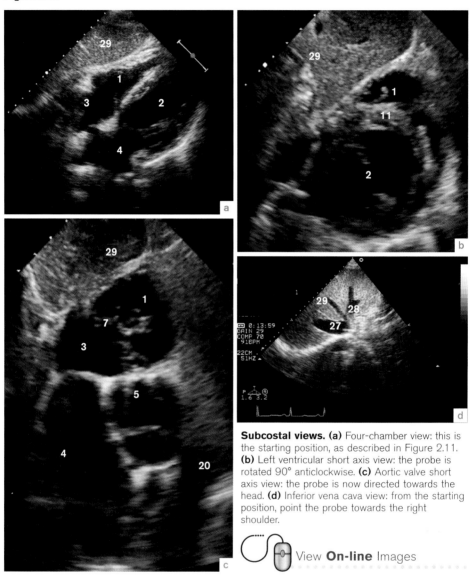

Subcostal views. (a) Four-chamber view: this is the starting position, as described in Figure 2.11. **(b)** Left ventricular short axis view: the probe is rotated 90° anticlockwise. **(c)** Aortic valve short axis view: the probe is now directed towards the head. **(d)** Inferior vena cava view: from the starting position, point the probe towards the right shoulder.

View **On-line** Images

Right parasternal view

This view is used specifically for interrogating the aortic valve and ascending aorta. It is well aligned with transaortic blood flow, and gives more accurate estimates of aortic valve gradient than apical views. The patient should be rolled on to the right-hand side to bring the heart and aorta forward (Fig. 2.15). The probe is placed in the second or third intercostal space.

Ideally a dedicated Doppler probe should be used, but alignment can be difficult because there is no two-dimensional image for guidance. If a standard

Figure 2.13

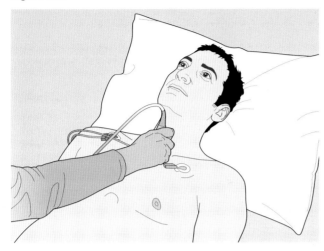

Suprasternal views. The patient is allowed to recline at 45° and tilt the head backwards. Position the probe in the suprasternal notch. Point the marker towards the left shoulder for views of the descending aorta, and to the right shoulder for the ascending aorta.

Figure 2.14

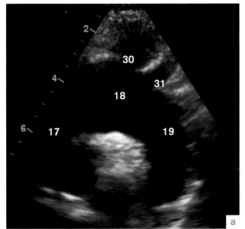 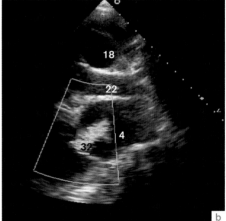

Suprasternal views. (a) Aortic arch and descending aorta. **(b)** Crab view of left atrium: the colour flow Doppler represents blood flow into the left atrium from the right inferior pulmonary vein.

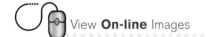 View **On-line** Images

multipurpose probe is used, the continuous wave Doppler cursor can be placed using CFM Doppler guidance (Fig. 2.16).

Putting it all together

A complete echo examination should use most, if not all, of these views in sequence. Each two-dimensional view instantly provides information about cardiac

Figure 2.15

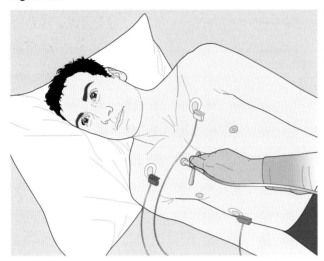

Right parasternal view. Roll the patient on to the right-hand side, to bring the heart and aorta forward. Position the stand-alone Doppler probe in the second or third right intercostal space. Make small adjustments in position to find transaortic flow.

Figure 2.16

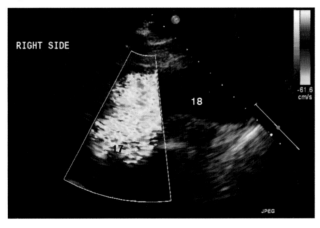

Right parasternal view. The ascending aorta and aortic arch are shown in this patient with severe aortic stenosis. Colour flow mapping Doppler shows a turbulent high-velocity jet arising from the aortic valve.

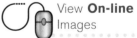 View **On-line** Images

structure and function, but in addition, all other available echo modalities (M-mode, Doppler, tissue Doppler) are required specifically to assess chamber dimensions, ventricular function, valvular function and blood flow. The routine views therefore provide the skeleton for the rest of the echo examination.

A comprehensive study can be quite daunting to begin with, so you need to gain confidence at doing the basics before you try anything complicated. As you make progress, build up your repertoire of views, modalities and techniques. Try to stick to a routine so that you never forget anything important. As you go along, identify all the structures you can see, and form an opinion about their appearance. By doing this you will quickly learn to discriminate between normal, and deviations from normal. You will also avoid missing things.

Optimising the picture

Picture quality is determined by many factors to do with the patient, the operator, the environment where the echo takes place and the settings of the echo machine. You should spend some time optimising as many factors as possible, as you will be rewarded with good images. Of course, some factors, such as poor echo windows, cannot be changed, leading to suboptimal picture quality, but even in these circumstances things can often be improved.

Patient optimisation

Before starting the examination, explain the nature of the procedure to the patient to ensure maximum cooperation and obtain consent. The patient's chest should be bare, and electrocardiograph (ECG) electrodes should be removed from the echo windows if these are present. Position the patient on the echo couch at 45°, rolled on to the left-hand side (left lateral decubitus position). Be prepared to adjust this position, as required, and make sure you have a comfortable position for yourself.

Images are often improved by asking patients to hold their breath in expiration, as this reduces lung volumes and decreases interference from respiratory movement.

A good ECG trace enhances image acquisition. ECG electrodes should be placed on each shoulder and one at the subcostal margin. The standard configuration of leads is ʀed/ʀight shoulder, yeʟʟow/ʟeft shoulder, green/costal margin. Sometimes better tracings are obtained if the yellow and green leads are swapped over. Usually a 1–2-beat recording is sufficient, but you should record at least 3 beats in patients with atrial fibrillation, frequent ectopics or tachycardia above 100 beats per minute (bpm).

Examination environment

The echo should be carried out in a dedicated room that is quiet and undisturbed. The lighting should be dimmed, and a special echo couch should be available, preferably with a cut-away section to facilitate apical imaging. Ultrasound gel is used sparingly to improve contact between transducer and skin.

Echo optimisation

Even the most basic echo machines allow some degree of control over ultrasound settings and image processing, and you should tailor these for every view on every patient. The main parameters to be adjusted depend on the mode in use.

Two-dimensional imaging

Probe choice

Echo machines often have several probes attached, so make sure you chose the right one. Probe choice is important because differences in frequency determine the maximum resolution and depth of ultrasound penetration. *Resolution* is the smallest distance between objects that can be detected by the ultrasound beam and is equivalent to the ultrasound wavelength. For example, a standard 3-MHz probe has a resolution of 0.5 mm in soft tissues. For the highest resolution, the shortest possible wavelength / highest-frequency probe should be used, but this will reduce tissue *penetration*. For this reason adult probes work around the 3-MHz range, whilst paediatric probes can use frequencies up to 8 MHz. In practice a standard multipurpose adult probe will suffice for the majority of adult echo examinations, unless the patient is particularly large or small.

Sector depth

Depth should be adjusted for each view so that the whole heart is displayed, with areas of interest in the centre of the picture, unless you need to concentrate on a specific structure. Setting the depth too low may lead to deep structures being missed, whilst a high setting may make the overall size of the heart too small for proper assessment (Fig. 3.1).

Sector width

Although using the maximum sector width will ensure visualisation of as much of the heart as possible, it is sometimes preferable to reduce it to include only those structures under scrutiny. This can improve image quality because the smaller sector can be scanned more times per second (increased frame rate) (Fig. 3.2).

Gain

Image brightness depends on the strength of the ultrasound signal received by the transducer. Signal strength depends predominantly on the distance travelled, but

Figure 3.1

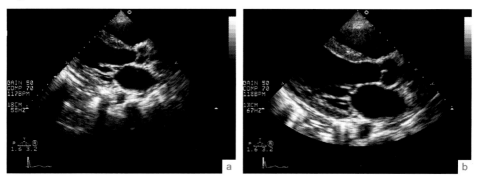

Adjusting depth setting. Parasternal long axis views. **(a)** Depth set to 17 cm. The heart is small in comparison to the sector. **(b)** Depth set to 13 cm. The heart fills the sector, with adequate visualisation of the posterior structures.

Figure 3.2

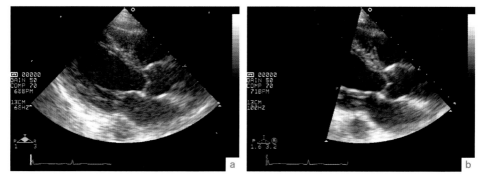

Sector width adjustment. (a, b) Parasternal long axis views. Narrowing the sector width around the aortic valve enhances the image quality, by increasing the frame rate.

is also affected by the reflective properties of the tissues encountered. The resulting image therefore tends to be brighter nearer the transducer. To produce a more homogeneous picture, weak signals can be amplified using time gain compensation (TGC), which boosts the intensity of later signals (more distant objects). TGCs can be used manually to adjust gain at specific depths. These are usually vertical slide controls on the control panel. In a similar manner lateral gain compensation (LGC) can used to amplify the signal from specific sectors of the image to compensate for edge drop-out (Fig. 3.3). Automatic gain optimisation is available on some echo machines.

Although a brighter picture may appear better, excessive gain can reduce the definition between structures and lead to artefact. A correctly adjusted image should have uniform intensity of solid structures, and a slight speckling of the blood-filled cavities.

Focusing

Ultrasound waves can be focused at a particular depth by controlling the sequence in which piezoelectric crystals are activated. The result is to concentrate the

Figure 3.3

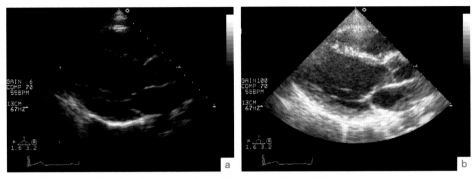

Gain adjustment. Parasternal long axis views. **(a)** Low overall gain. **(b)** Excessive overall gain.

Figure 3.4

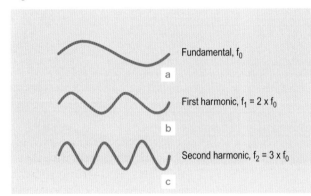

Fundamental, f₀

a

First harmonic, f₁ = 2 x f₀

b

Second harmonic, f₂ = 3 x f₀

c

Principles of harmonics. The lines represent a string of an instrument which vibrates to produce a sound wave. **(a)** At the fundamental frequency the wavelength of the emitted sound is equal to the length of the string. **(b)** The second harmonic has a frequency double that of the fundamental, and half its wavelength. **(c)** The next harmonic has a frequency of three times the fundamental. Similar principles apply to ultrasound harmonics.

ultrasound signal in a small area, thereby enhancing the intensity of the reflected signal. Focus depth should be adjusted to just below the structure of interest, and readjusted as required for each view.

Harmonics

Tissue harmonic imaging (THI) is a setting used to enhance picture quality. The concept of harmonics will be familiar to musicians as the relationship between notes separated by octaves. For example, if a guitar string is plucked it sounds a particular note that has a specific fundamental frequency (f_0) related to the length of the string (Fig. 3.4). This is the frequency at which the string will resonate. The note an octave above this has a frequency double that of the fundamental (first harmonic), and further octaves are multiples of the fundamental frequency (second harmonic, and so on). The fundamental frequency alone can sound quite bland and hollow, and usually a musical note comprises a mixture of the fundamental and harmonics, which give the note its tone quality and interest.

Figure 3.5

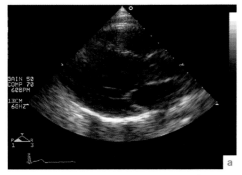
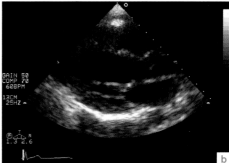
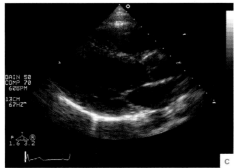

Harmonics. Parasternal long axis views.
(a) Fundamental imaging: image is grainy. **(b)** First harmonic: the image is grainy but the myocardial definition is enhanced. **(c)** Second harmonic: improved image quality.

In a similar manner ultrasound waves consist of a fundamental frequency determined by the construction of the transducer. When ultrasound interacts with tissue, causing it to vibrate, harmonics are generated that are multiples of the fundamental frequency. This feature of ultrasound behaviour is useful because the fundamental frequency is rapidly attenuated as it penetrates tissue, whereas the harmonic frequencies actually become stronger within a range of 4–8 cm from the transducer. THI is a method of selectively using the harmonic frequencies whilst suppressing the fundamental, resulting in enhanced far field picture quality (Fig. 3.5). It also avoids near field artefacts that can occur with fundamental imaging.

In general, higher THI settings improve image quality, but highly reflective structures such as valves and pericardium appear thicker than they actually are.

Colour flow mapping Doppler

Sector size

The colour flow mapping (CFM) Doppler sector should be positioned over the structure of interest. For regurgitant jets you should aim to include the whole jet, as well as the zone of flow convergence before the valve, if present. Although a large sector is preferable, it can slow down image processing and impair overall image quality. This can be minimised by blanking out the two-dimensional imaging sector either side of the CFM sector using the black and white suppress option available on many echo machines.

Figure 3.6

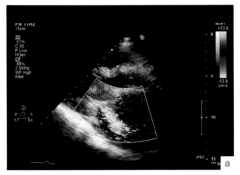

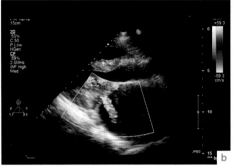

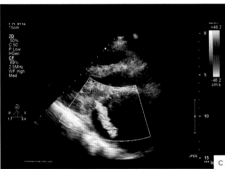

Optimising colour flow mapping (CFM) Doppler. Parasternal long axis views. **(a)** High CFM gain setting. **(b)** Low gain setting. **(c)** Low aliasing velocity. The apparent size of a regurgitant jet can be altered by the settings of the CFM Doppler. High gain increases the area of the jet and low gain reduces this. A low aliasing velocity also tends to increase the jet area.

Colour gain

Doppler colour flow signals can be amplified using the gain control to enhance detection of small jets of abnormal flow. However, it is very important that this is set correctly as it will affect the apparent severity of regurgitant valve lesions. The optimal level of gain usually causes a minute amount of speckling. Excessive gain will lead to artefact, and suppressed gain reduces the size of regurgitant jets and misses subtle abnormalities of flow (Fig. 3.6).

Aliasing velocity

The velocity range of CFM is indicated on a scale at the side of the display, and is usually set automatically. The velocities at which aliasing occurs are defined by the limits of the scale, and adjusting this will alter the appearance of blood flow, particularly regurgitant jets (Fig. 3.6). This needs to be taken into account when interpreting severity of regurgitation. Techniques such as proximal isovelocity surface area (PISA) require specific aliasing velocities, as well as adjustment of the baseline to enhance colour contrast (see later chapters).

Spectral Doppler

Type of Doppler

The choice of spectral Doppler mode depends on the specific application and the likely velocity range required: standard applications are dealt with in later chapters

Figure 3.7

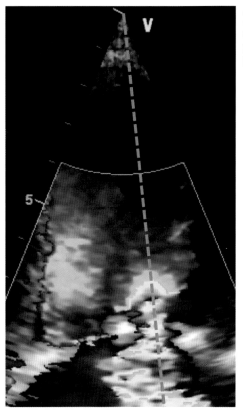

Alignment of spectral Doppler. Apical four-chamber view. In this example of mitral regurgitation the Doppler cursor is aligned with the portion of the regurgitant jet (vena contracta) as it passes through the valve orifice.

on assessing valvular lesions. In general, pulse wave Doppler should be used where measurement of velocity at a precise location is required, whilst continuous wave Doppler is used where high velocities are expected.

Position of sample volume/cursor

The sample volume/cursor should be positioned anatomically using two-dimensional echo. In addition CFM should be used to ensure proper alignment with blood flow. If the angle between the Doppler cursor and blood flow is greater than 20°, peak velocities will be underestimated. For regurgitant jets, the cursor should pass through the narrow portion of the jet, just after the valve orifice, known as the vena contracta (Fig. 3.7).

Scale/baseline

The scale and baseline of the spectral display should be adjusted to show the feature of interest in maximal detail, allowing precise measurements (Fig. 3.8).

Figure 3.8

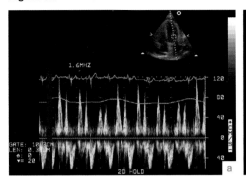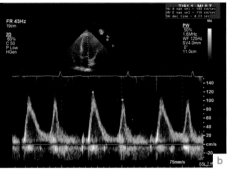

Optimisation of spectral Doppler. Transmitral pulse wave Doppler recordings. **(a)** The scan speed has been set to 25 mm/s to allow the respiratory variation in mitral inflow velocity to be better appreciated in this case of cardiac tamponade. **(b)** The faster scan speed in this case (75 mm/s) allows the individual components of transmitral flow to be analysed in detail. Note also that the baseline and scale of the recordings have been adjusted to display the Doppler readings optimally.

Sweep speed

The time scale of spectral Doppler can be altered according to the application (Fig. 3.8). The standard sweep speed is 50 mm/s, and will usually suffice: increased sweep speeds stretch out the signals, so that accurate time measurements can be made. Alternatively, slower sweep speeds compress multiple cardiac cycles together, allowing assessment of respiratory variation over several seconds.

CHAPTER

4

The left ventricle

The anatomy of the left ventricle

The left ventricle is a thick-walled chamber that is shaped rather like one end of a rugby ball. At the base is the mitral valve, and the left ventricular outflow tract, from which blood enters and leaves the left ventricle. It has few trabeculations and is therefore smooth-walled. There are two groups of papillary muscles that support the mitral valve apparatus and insert into the left ventricular free wall. The interventricular septum is defined by the attachment of the right ventricular free walls to the left ventricle.

The muscle fibres of the left ventricular wall are arranged in a complex spiral pattern from base to apex that varies with depth within the wall. Fibres are generally arranged circumferentially in the mid-wall, and more longitudinally in the subendocardium and subepicardium. This gives the heart a twisting motion during contraction, rather than a uniform shortening.

Echocardiographic appearance

The left ventricle is a feature of almost all standard echocardiographic views, and is particularly well seen on the parasternal long axis (PSLAX), parasternal short axis (PSSAX), apical four-, three- and two-chamber (A4C, A3C and A2C) views (Figs 2.5, 2.8, 2.10 and 2.12). Complete assessment of left ventricular structure and function requires many different views, and should be covered by a routine echo examination.

The echo density of normal myocardium should be slightly less than that of the valves or pericardium. Wall thickness should be uniform, though in elderly patients isolated hypertrophy of the proximal septum can occur (Fig. 4.1). This is a normal variant and is rarely of any significance.

Figure 4.1

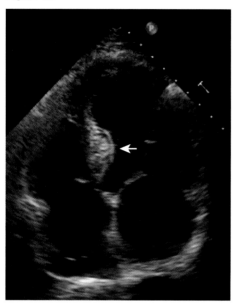

Proximal septal hypertrophy. Apical four-chamber view. There is proximal septal hypertrophy, with localised thickening of the basal region of the interventricular septum (arrow). The remainder of the left ventricular wall has normal thickness.

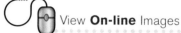
View **On-line** Images

Left ventricular chords are thin fibrous strings that are occasionally seen crossing the ventricular cavity, either from the free wall to the septum (Fig. 4.2) or run along the length of a wall. They are echo-bright, and share a similar appearance to chordae of the mitral valve. They appear to tighten and slacken with the cardiac cycle.

Left ventricular structure

The standard left ventricular dimensions include interventricular septal (IVS) wall thickness, left ventricular internal diameter (LVID) and posterior wall thickness (PWT) at end diastole and systole (Fig. 4.3). These measurements provide important information about left ventricular structure, and can also be used to calculate parameters such as left ventricular mass and fractional shortening. Assessment of left ventricular volumes will be covered in a later section.

The usual approach is to use two-dimensional imaging from the PSLAX view to guide placement of the M-mode cursor across the left ventricular chamber at the level of the mitral valve tips. The cursor must be aligned perpendicular to the left ventricular long axis; otherwise dimensions will be overestimated. If proper alignment cannot be achieved it is recommended that direct measurements are made from the two-dimensional images (Fig. 4.3). Measurements should be made directly from the borders of the left ventricular walls, avoiding structures such as papillary muscle/mitral valve chordae.

To account for variation caused by differences in body size it is recommended that chamber dimensions and volumes are normalised to body surface area and

Figure 4.2

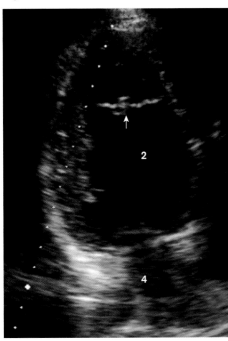

Left ventricular chord. Apical four-chamber view. A chord (arrow) traverses the left ventricular cavity from the free wall to the septum.

2

4

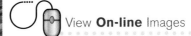 View **On-line** Images

gender. Indexed and gender-specific values are given for all dimensions/volumes in Appendix 1.

Left ventricular mass

A variety of methods can be used to estimate left ventricular mass. In practice it is only necessary to know the measurements required, as most echo software packages will automatically calculate left ventricular mass from the relevant data. The formulae are quoted in Appendix 2 for those who wish to know.

These formulae assume left ventricular geometry is symmetrical (e.g. concentric left ventricular hypertrophy: LVH), but become inaccurate as soon as geometry is distorted or asymmetric (e.g. remodelling after myocardial infarction).

M-mode methods

Left ventricular wall thickness

IVS thickness or PWT can be measured in diastole from M-mode recordings in the PSLAX view. More than 1.0 cm is considered abnormal in adult men, and >0.9 cm in adult women. Ranges of abnormality are given in Appendix 1. If the left ventricle is dilated, overall left ventricular mass may be increased despite apparently normal wall thickness, so this simple approach has obvious limitations.

Figure 4.3

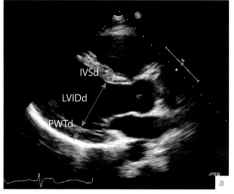
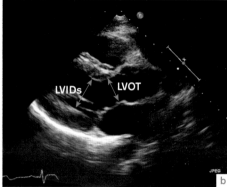

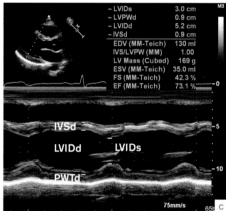

– LVIDs	3.0 cm
– LVPWd	0.9 cm
– LVIDd	5.2 cm
– IVSd	0.9 cm
EDV (MM-Teich)	130 ml
IVS/LVPW (MM)	1.00
LV Mass (Cubed)	169 g
ESV (MM-Teich)	35.0 ml
FS (MM-Teich)	42.3 %
EF (MM-Teich)	73.1 %

Left ventricular dimensions. (a) Parasternal long axis (PSLAX) view, end diastole. **(b)** PSLAX view, end systole. **(c)** M-mode. IVSd, diastolic interventricular septal thickness; LVIDd, diastolic left ventricular internal diameter; LVIDs, systolic left ventricular diameter; PWTd, diastolic posterior wall thickness; LVOT, left ventricular outflow tract.

Cubed formula

This assumes that the left ventricle is shaped like the end of a rugby ball (prolate ellipsoid). You simply need to measure three things (IVSd, LVIDd and PWTd), as illustrated in Figure 4.3c.

Two-dimensional methods

Area–length formula

This formula requires three simple measurements (Fig. 4.4):

1. The length of the left ventricle (L) from the endocardial surface of the apex to the midpoint of the mitral annulus.
2. The area defined by the epicardial surface of the left ventricle in diastole in a PSSAX view at the level of the papillary muscles (A_1).
3. The area defined by the endocardial surface of the left ventricular cavity in the same view (A_2). Do not include the papillary muscles in the measurement.

Figure 4.4

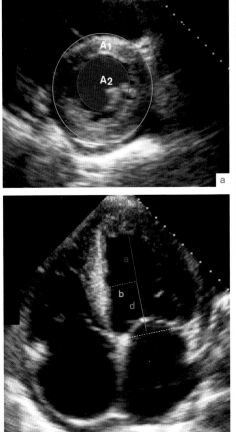

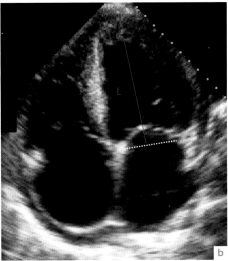

Left ventricular mass: two-dimensional methods. (a) Parasternal short axis (PSSAX) view: papillary level. **(b** and **c)** Apical four-chamber view. *Area–length method:* trace the area of the epicardial (A₁) and endocardial borders (A₂) from the PSSAX view at end diastole. The difference between these reflects the area of myocardium. Next, measure the length (L) of the left ventricle from the apex to the midpoint of the mitral valve annulus plane. *Truncated ellipsoid method:* determine A₁ and A₂ as above. The length of the left ventricle is subdivided into an apical portion (a) and a basal portion (d). The subdivision is made at the widest minor axis radius (b). Dimension b is calculated from the area data and does not need to be measured directly.

Truncated ellipsoid

Essentially this requires very similar measurements to the area–length method (Fig. 4.4): A_1 and A_2 are measured as before. The length L is subdivided into lengths a and d at the point where the diameter of the left ventricle is maximal: a is the length from the apex to the intersection of the maximal minor axis and d is the length from this intersection to the midpoint of the mitral annular plane.

Left ventricular hypertrophy

LVH is defined as an increase in the mass of the left ventricle due to enlargement of the muscle cells, and extracellular fibrosis. It can occur as a primary condition (e.g. hypertrophic cardiomyopathy) or secondary to pathologies such as hypertension, myocardial infarction and valvular heart disease. Different patterns of LVH occur in the context of specific pathologies: concentric LVH typically occurs in response to pressure overload (e.g. aortic stenosis or hypertension) and results in symmetrical hypertrophy that encroaches on left ventricular internal diameter, leading to a reduced cavity size. Eccentric hypertrophy occurs in volume overload (e.g. aortic or mitral regurgitation), whereby left ventricular mass increases without a reduction in left ventricular diameter.

Left ventricular systolic function

Assessment of left ventricular function is the most frequent reason for performing an echo, and yet it is notoriously difficult to master. Some of the difficulty relates to the technical aspects of echo, but there are also other problems that apply universally to all methods of assessing left ventricular function.

First of all, the left ventricle is a complex pump that continually cycles between systole and diastole: it is never in a fixed state. Not surprisingly, there is no single parameter that can be measured that takes into account all phases of the cardiac cycle. Secondly, cardiac function automatically adjusts to the prevailing haemodynamic conditions, so that cardiac output varies according to the filling pressure of the left ventricle (preload) and the resistance that has to be pumped against (afterload) (Fig. 4.5). This is the Frank–Starling mechanism, and all measures of left ventricular function, whether echocardiographic or not, are influenced by this to a greater or lesser degree. Finally, left ventricular function or shape is often distorted in a regionalised manner, and this adds to the complexity of assessing function.

Figure 4.5

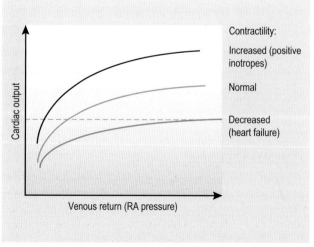

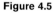

Frank–Starling mechanism. The Frank–Starling mechanism describes the variation of cardiac output with preload: as preload increases, cardiac output also increases in a non-linear manner, eventually reaching a plateau. Different contractile states are depicted, and it can be seen that the relationship between cardiac output and preload is much flatter in cardiac failure. It is also evident that an identical cardiac output can be achieved in each contractile state with different preloads (dashed line). Red line, heart failure; blue line, normal cardiac systolic function; black line, increased cardiac contractility due to inotropes. RA, right atrial.

What is the best measure of left ventricular function?

Assessment of left ventricular function can be as complex or simple as you wish to make it. The large number of methods that have been described reflects the fact that all of them have problems. In current clinical practice almost all decisions rely on the assessment of left ventricular ejection fraction (EF) and detection of regional wall motion abnormalities. Although these parameters are not perfect, it is sensible to concentrate on these aspects of the echo examination, rather than other parameters that are less relevant clinically.

Subjective assessment

It is common practice to grade global left ventricular systolic function by 'eyeball' into broad categories of normal function, or mild, moderate and severe impairment. To do this accurately you need to be experienced, and you should spend time reviewing all the echo movies in Chapter 2 to get a feel for normal left ventricular function.

You will notice that contraction causes thickening of the myocardium, as well as inward displacement. Thickening by more than 30% is considered normal (Fig. 4.6a and b), and it is a far better indicator of contraction than movement *per se*. Movement of a myocardial segment can be misleading because it can be dragged by adjacent contracting segments, or move simply because of respiration. Thickening less than 30% indicates hypokinesis, whilst absence of thickening defines akinesis (Fig. 4.6c–f). Dyskinetic segments demonstrate paradoxical outward movement during systole (Fig. 4.6g and h), which may reflect complete absence of contractile function. However, IVS dyskinesia can also occur with left bundle branch block, right ventricular pacing, right ventricular pressure overload, pericardial constriction and following cardiac surgery. The significance of dyskinesis is therefore subject to the clinical context of the patient.

There are several potential pitfalls to bear in mind when assessing left ventricular function. First, no single echocardiographic view reflects the overall function of the heart because regional differences may exist. Multiple views are therefore required to assess all the regions of the left ventricle, many of which may not be easily visualised in every patient. Sometimes the myocardium can appear hypokinetic in one view, but not in others. This is particularly common with the apical views because the apex can be difficult to visualise, and detection of thickening in the transverse plane can be poor. Furthermore, the arrangement of myocardial fibres in the left ventricle is complex and contraction does not simply lead to radial shortening, but also longitudinal and torsional movement, which is difficult to appreciate by eye.

Certain situations can lead to an overestimate of left ventricular function and caution should be exercised. Oblique views can cause foreshortening, so that the ventricle appears small and wall motion is exaggerated. This is a particular problem with apical views, and can be avoided by constant attention to maintaining the maximal ventricular size. Severe mitral regurgitation can also 'flatter' the appearance of left ventricular function despite significant impairment, as blood is easily offloaded into the left atrium, rather than into the systemic circulation.

Figure 4.6

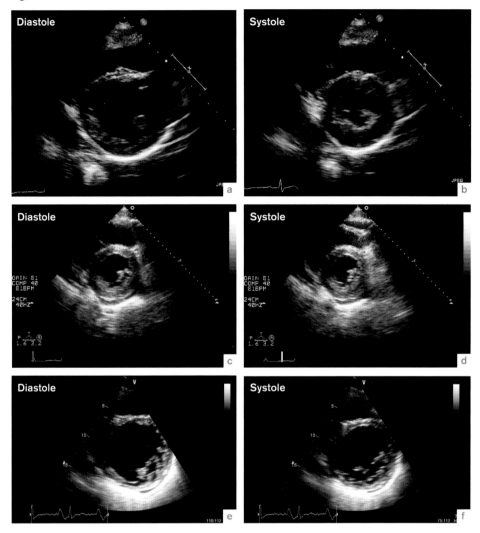

Semiquantitative assessment

Regional differences in left ventricular function often arise in the presence of ischaemic heart disease because the coronary arteries supply distinct territories of myocardium. Impairment or occlusion of the blood supply in one artery will lead to contractile abnormalities in that territory, but others will be unaffected. Such variations are referred to as regional wall motion abnormalities (RWMAs).

To take account of RWMAs, scoring systems have been developed that divide the left ventricle up into distinct segments, reflecting the coronary blood supply. This allows a more quantitative assessment of left ventricular function than is possible by purely subjective assessment. The left ventricle is divided into thirds

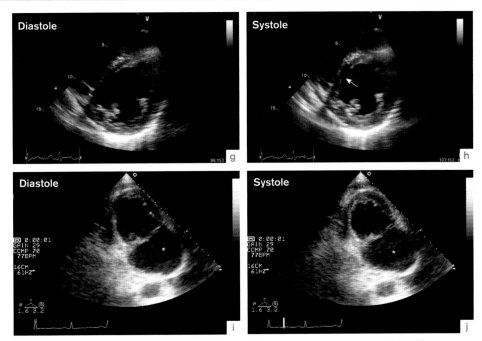

Visual assessment of left ventricular systolic function. Parasternal short axis (PSSAX) views. **(a** and **b)** Normal function. Significant thickening of all myocardial segments is seen during systole, indicating normal contractile function. **(c** and **d)** Hypokinesis. There is reduced thickening in all segments. **(e** and **f)** Akinesis. Previous myocardial infarction has caused anteroseptal and anterior akinesis. **(g** and **h)** Dyskinesis. Note the outward movement of the septum during systole (arrow). **(i** and **j)** Aneurysm. Note the aneurysm of the inferior wall (*).

View **On-line** Images

(apical, mid and basal) along its long axis, and subdivided into segments. The mid and basal portions have six segments, arranged around the short axis circumference, whilst the apical portion has only four segments (Fig. 4.7). This is therefore described as a 16-segment model. The function of each segment is scored in a standardised manner according to the principles described in Table 4.1.

The wall motion score index (WMSI) is the sum of scores divided by the number of segments evaluated. By definition a normal ventricle has a score of 1, whilst a score above 1 indicates left ventricular impairment. Although WMSI correlates with EF it is not possible to give corresponding values for each. You should review the echo movies from Figure 4.6 and identify and score the segments in each case. Most echo reporting packages will allow you to report wall motion scores and will calculate WMSI automatically.

A 17-segment model is recommended by the American Society of Echocardiography as this provides the best agreement with anatomical data and allows conformity with other imaging modalities such as cardiac magnetic resonance imaging and nuclear perfusion imaging. This model has an extra segment that is formed by the cap of the apex, and has no endocardial border (Fig. 4.7b). Although

Figure 4.7

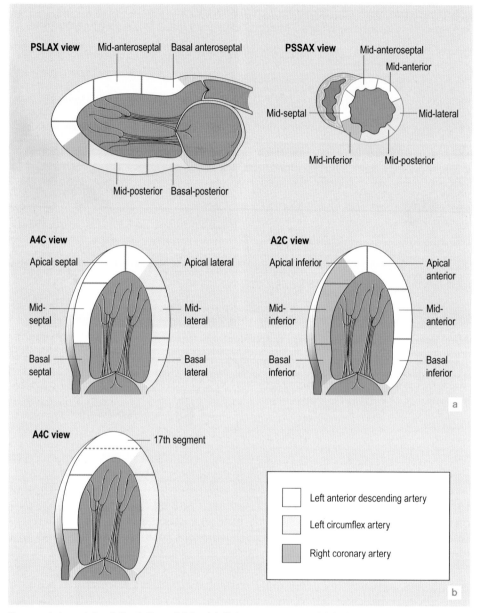

Segmental models of the left ventricle. (a) Sixteen-segment model. In the standard parasternal and apical views the left ventricle can be divided into 16 segments that can be scored individually for myocardial function. Coronary arterial blood supply is indicated by the colour of the segments, though considerable variation exists between individuals. Yellow, left anterior descending artery; orange, right coronary artery; green, left circumflex artery. **(b)** Seventeen-segment model. An additional apical segment is illustrated in the apical four-chamber (A4C) view. The terminology for individual segments also differs from the 16-segment model. PSLAX, parasternal long axis; PSSAX, parasternal short axis; A2C, apical two-chamber.

Table 4.1 Wall motion scoring criteria

Score	Description	Comments
1	Normal	Normal inward movement and myocardial thickening >30%
2	Hypokinetic	Reduced movement and thickening <30%
3	Akinetic	Absent thickening
4	Dyskinetic	Paradoxical outward movement during systole
5	Aneurysmal	Diastolic wall deformity: myocardium thinned and hyperreflectant

standardisation between techniques is helpful for comparison, the 17th segment can only be properly assessed by perfusion techniques and so is not necessarily relevant to non-contrast-enhanced transthoracic echocardiography.

Quantitative assessment

Fractional shortening

This is simply the fractional change in left ventricular diameter during systole compared to diastole. It is a reliable measure of left ventricular function as long as there are no RWMAs. To perform this measurement you need to determine end diastolic diameter (LVIDd) and end systolic diameter (LVIDs) from M-mode measurements of the basal segments of the left ventricle in PSLAX view (Fig. 4.3c).

$$\text{Fractional shortening} = \frac{\text{LVIDd} - \text{LVIDs}}{\text{LVIDd}} \times 100$$

Sex-specific normal ranges are given in Appendix 1. Generally, normal fractional shortening is 26–44%.

Clearly, this model assumes that the basal segments adequately reflect global left ventricular function. This is only likely to be true when cardiac function is completely normal, or there is global left ventricular dysfunction. In any other situations a more complex method should be used to assess left ventricular function.

Ejection fraction

The most commonly used measure of cardiac function is the left ventricular EF. This is simply the proportion of blood pumped out of the left ventricle during each cardiac cycle. Therefore to calculate EF we have to estimate the volume of the left ventricle at the end of diastole and systole.

$$\text{Ejection fraction (\%)} = \frac{\text{Stroke volume}}{\text{End diastolic volume}} \times 100$$

$$\text{Stroke volume} = \text{end diastolic volume} - \text{end systolic volume}$$

Accepted normal ranges are given in Table 4.2 and Appendix 1.

Table 4.2 Ejection fraction

Ejection fraction (%)	Left ventricular systolic function
55–85	Normal
45–54	Mild impairment
30–44	Moderate impairment
<30	Severe impairment

Figure 4.8

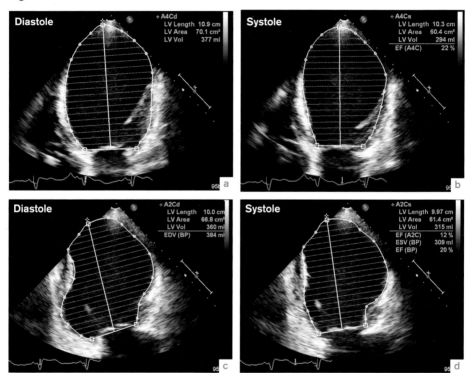

Determination of ejection fraction: modified Simpson's rule. Ejection fraction can be estimated from biplane measurements of left ventricular shape in end diastole (**a** and **c**) and end systole (**b** and **d**). This allows calculation of left ventricular volumes and hence ejection fraction. In this case ejection fraction was calculated as 20% (normal 55–85%).

View **On-line** Images

A number of methods have been described which extrapolate volumes from single measurements of the ventricular diameter, or multiple measurements in more than one plane. Currently the recommended method is the biplane modified Simpson's rule. This attempts to take account of irregular ventricular geometry or regional wall motion abnormalities, by measuring left ventricular cavity area in two planes perpendicular to each other. Left ventricular volume is then calculated by dividing the cavity into 20 small cylinders of equal height, stacked together like a pile of coins. The left ventricular volume is the sum of the individual cylinder volumes (Fig. 4.8).

To use this method, trace the endocardial border in systole and diastole in A4C and A2C views (these are perpendicular to each other): most echo software packages will automatically subdivide the traced areas into slices and calculate volumes for each, and overall ejection fraction.

Obviously this method is still not perfect because only two planes are analysed, and regional abnormalities in other planes are not taken into account. For example, a posterior wall aneurysm will not be included in either A4C or A2C views, but obviously will have a significant effect on left ventricular performance. Furthermore, it is critically dependent on identification of endocardial borders, which may not always be well defined. Advanced echo technologies, such as three-dimensional echo, automatic edge detection software and left ventricular contrast agents, offer some hope of circumventing these limitations (see Chapter 21).

Reporting box

Reporting left ventricular (LV) function

Summary

- Comment on global systolic and diastolic function

Qualitative data

- Regional wall motion abnormalities
- Regions of scar, aneurysm, hypertrophy

Quantitative data

- LV dimensions
- Fractional shortening
- LV volumes
- Ejection fraction
- LV mass
- E:A ratio
- Deceleration time
- E:Ea ratio

Diastolic function and dyssynchrony

Left ventricular diastolic function

Diastolic function is the ability of the left ventricle to fill with blood from the left atrium. It is determined largely by left ventricular relaxation, left ventricular stiffness (compliance), and to a lesser extent, left atrial function.

Assessment of diastolic filling requires an understanding of the four phases of diastole:

1. *Isovolumic relaxation*. Diastole begins with the onset of left ventricular relaxation and is marked by closure of the aortic valve. During this initial period of relaxation, left ventricular pressure falls rapidly. Both the aortic and mitral valves are closed, so the volume of the left ventricle does not change.

2. *Early rapid filling*. The next phase occurs when left ventricular pressure falls to below that of the left atrium, allowing the mitral valve to open. Blood passively enters the left ventricle from the left atrium due to the small pressure gradient between them. Usually this accounts for the majority of left ventricular filling, in terms of volume and velocity of blood flow.

3. *Diastasis*. During this phase passive low-velocity filling occurs. The gradient between the left atrium and ventricle is minimal.

4. *Late filling*. The final phase occurs with atrial contraction, which actively pumps blood across the mitral valve, contributing 20–30% of left ventricular filling.

Diastolic dysfunction

Diastolic dysfunction occurs when there is a problem with myocardial relaxation and/or stiffness. Ultimately this translates into an increase in left ventricular and left atrial diastolic pressures, which in turn impacts on the pulmonary circulation. These changes in pressure mean that the pattern of blood flow into the left ventricle is altered in terms of timing, duration and velocity. It is these changes that can be detected by echocardiographic assessment.

Conditions associated with diastolic dysfunction

Diastolic dysfunction can occur in isolation, often as part of the natural ageing process, or associated with left ventricular hypertrophy. In some studies around 50% of patients with a clinical diagnosis of heart failure have a normal ejection fraction but abnormal diastolic function: this is known as heart failure with preserved ejection fraction.

A wide range of conditions are associated with diastolic dysfunction: left ventricular hypertrophy (usually due to hypertension), ischaemic heart disease and dilated cardiomyopathy are some of the more common ones. By definition restrictive cardiomyopathy is associated with severe diastolic dysfunction. In most cases there is significant left atrial dilatation by virtue of the fact that left atrial pressure is chronically increased.

Pulse wave Doppler assessment of diastolic function

The phases of transmitral blood flow can be demonstrated using pulse wave (PW) Doppler (Fig. 5.1). This requires an apical four-chamber (A4C) view with the PW sample volume placed at the level of the mitral valve tips.

The typical pattern shows an E wave corresponding to the early filling phase, followed by an A wave of lower velocity which occurs with atrial contraction. A large number of parameters of the E and A waves can be measured to assess left ventricular diastolic function, but in practice only a limited number are needed routinely (Fig. 5.1): E wave peak velocity (E), A wave peak velocity (A), E:A ratio, A wave duration and E wave deceleration time (DT). If the sample volume is not correctly positioned the absolute velocities recorded will be altered, but the relative E:A pattern will still be preserved.

As diastolic function deteriorates, left ventricular end diastolic pressure increases, which in turn causes an increase in left atrial pressure, altering the pattern of blood flow between left atrium and left ventricle. Four patterns of diastolic function can be recognised from mitral valve inflow Doppler signals (Fig. 5.1):

1. *Normal.* Early passive filling predominates in terms of volume and velocity (E>A wave velocity).
2. *Impaired relaxation.* Left ventricular relaxation occurs during the early phase of diastole. If relaxation is impaired and prolonged, early passive filling of the left ventricle is affected, resulting in greater dependence on atrial contraction for filling. In other words, left ventricular filling is delayed, but left atrial pressure remains normal. This change in blood flow is

Figure 5.1

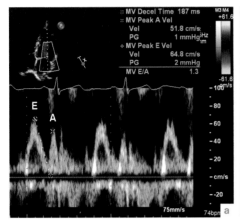

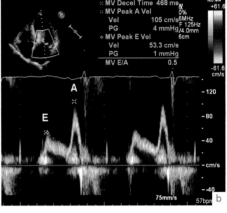

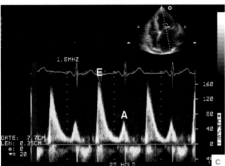

Patterns of transmitral flow. (a) Normal or pseudonormal filling pattern: E:A ratio 0.8–1.5. **(b)** Impaired relaxation: E:A reversal. **(c)** Restrictive filling pattern: E≫A.

reflected in a reduced E wave peak velocity, prolonged deceleration time and an increased A wave peak velocity (E<A wave velocity).

3. *Pseudonormal filling.* More severe diastolic dysfunction leads to a compensatory increase in left atrial pressure, which improves early passive filling, so that E wave peak velocity again predominates (E>A wave velocity).

4. *Restrictive filling.* In extreme cases the left ventricle may be so stiff that filling can only occur with very high left atrial pressure. A small increase in left ventricular volume results in a rapid and severe increase in left ventricular pressure and further filling is curtailed. Filling is therefore confined to the early phase of diastole, with very little flow occurring later. This pattern of flow is reflected in a high E wave peak velocity, rapid deceleration time and a small A wave peak velocity (E≫A wave velocity).

These patterns of blood flow provide a simple classification for left ventricular diastolic function, though there are certain caveats. First of all it is impossible to use this classification if atrial fibrillation is present due to the absence of the A wave. Furthermore, the classification is only valid in the presence of left ventricular systolic dysfunction, so abnormal diastolic patterns may occur in healthy youngsters (<50 years old) with completely normal systolic and diastolic function.

Diastolic filling is also influenced by heart rate and cannot be interpreted at rates greater than 100 beats per minute (bpm).

Although normal and pseudonormal filling patterns appear to be indistinguishable, in practice pseudonormal filling will invariably be associated with structural abnormalities such as left ventricular hypertrophy and atrial enlargement.

Doppler tissue imaging (DTI)

The principles behind DTI have been described in Chapter 1. This technique measures the velocity (not distance) of myocardial wall movement at a specific site, and is therefore more sensitive and specific for diastolic dysfunction than the PW Doppler methods described above.

The DTI sampling volume is positioned at the lateral or septal mitral valve annulus in the A4C view, with minimal angulation between the ultrasound beam and the plane of annular excursion (Fig. 5.2). As one would expect, there is inward acceleration/deceleration as myocardial contraction progresses (S wave). In diastole this is reversed as early passive ventricular filling and then atrial contraction occur: these velocity changes generate e' (e prime) and a' (a prime) waves, analogous to the E and A waves of transmitral blood flow. In general, septal peak velocities are lower than those at the lateral annulus, and e' decreases with age whilst a' increases.

Assessment of diastolic function with DTI requires the measurement of peak diastolic velocities at both the septal and lateral mitral valve annulus. Usually the average is used to give a global estimate of diastolic function. Diastolic dysfunction is associated with reduced e' velocities (septal e' <8 cm/s, lateral e' <10 cm/s): the lower the velocity, the worse the dysfunction.

In the context of abnormal left ventricular systolic function, left ventricular filling pressure correlates closely with the ratio of transmitral E wave peak velocity and average annular e' velocity (E/e' ratio). Normal filling pressure is predicted by E/e' <8, whereas a value >13 is highly suggestive of elevated left atrial pressure

Figure 5.2

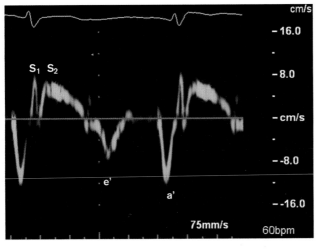

Left ventricular spectral pulse wave Doppler tissue imaging. S_1 and S_2, systolic velocities; e', early diastolic wave; a', late diastolic wave.

Figure 5.3

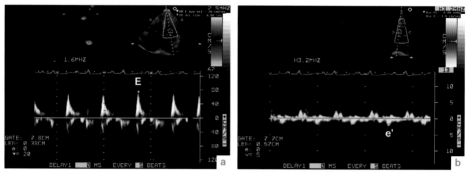

Assessing left ventricular filling pressure. (a) Transmitral filling pattern demonstrates a restrictive pattern. E peak velocity is 76 cm/s. **(b)** Tissue Doppler at the lateral mitral annulus demonstrates very low systolic and diastolic tissue velocities. e' is 1.9. Therefore E:e' is 40, suggesting the left ventricular filling pressure is markedly elevated.

Figure 5.4

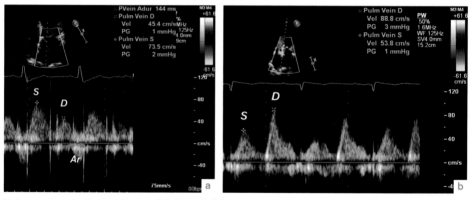

Pulmonary vein flow patterns. (a) Normal; **(b)** diastolic dominant flow. *S*, Systolic flow; *D*, diastolic flow; *Ar*, reverse atrial flow.

(Fig. 5.3). Between 8 and 13 other parameters need to be assessed to reach a conclusion about diastolic function.

Unfortunately the E/e' ratio is not universally applicable in all situations: it is most reliable if there is left ventricular systolic impairment. Caution is required if left ventricular systolic function is normal, or if there is significant annular calcification. Other diseases that can alter transmitral blood flow (e.g. mitral valve disease or pericardial constriction) may also give misleading E/e' ratios.

Pulmonary vein flow

Pulmonary vein flow is measured in the A4C view: continuous flow mapping is used to identify the right superior or inferior pulmonary vein, and a PW Doppler sample volume is positioned at least 0.5 cm within the vein (Fig. 5.4). It is important to adjust the depth settings to make sure that only one sample volume is present.

Normal pulmonary vein flow is complex, comprising a pulse of forward flow during ventricular systole (S wave), a pulse of forward flow in diastole (D wave), with a final small pulse of retrograde flow during atrial contraction (Ar wave). Forward flow occurs predominantly in systole, so the S wave peak velocity and velocity time integral (VTI) equals or exceeds that of the D wave.

Standard measurements include the peak velocities of the S, D and Ar waves, VTI of the S and D waves and the duration of the Ar wave. Important parameters of diastolic function are:

- The ratio of S and D wave peak velocities (normal >1)
- The systolic filling fraction. This is the systolic VTI as a percentage of total systolic and diastolic VTI (normal >40%)
- Ar duration – mitral A wave duration (normal <30 ms)

Of these, Ar–A duration ≥30 ms seems to be the most reliable as an indicator of raised left ventricular end diastolic pressure, irrespective of the underlying pathology. Reduced systolic forward flow (S:D ratio <1, systolic filling fraction <40%) is an indicator of diastolic dysfunction and raised left atrial pressure, but is less relevant with normal left ventricular systolic function, hypertrophic cardiomyopathy, mitral valve disease and atrial fibrillation.

Classifying diastolic function

A variety of classifications of diastolic function have been proposed: a simplified scheme based on the recommendations of the American Society of Echocardiography is indicated in Figure 5.5.

Four parameters need to be assessed for this classification:

1. Left atrial volume
2. Doppler tissue imaging
3. Transmitral PW Doppler
4. Pulmonary vein PW Doppler

Diastolic dysfunction is initially defined by the presence of significant left atrial enlargement (in the absence of other potential causes) and abnormal DTI values. Transmitral flow parameters are then used to classify the grade of dysfunction: impaired relaxation is grade 1, pseudonormal is grade 2 and restrictive is grade 3. Pulmonary vein flow, particularly abnormal Ar–A duration, can help to confirm significant diastolic dysfunction.

Ventricular synchrony

In the normal heart, rapid propagation of electrical impulses results in almost simultaneous contraction of all regions of the left and right ventricles. However, patients with advanced heart failure often have uncoordinated contraction, which may contribute to the poor performance of the heart. In selected patients biventricular pacing (also known as cardiac resynchronisation therapy, CRT) can restore

Figure 5.5

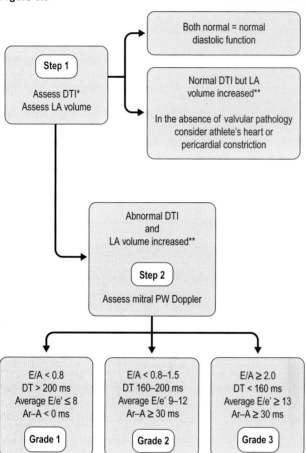

Classification of diastolic function. DTI, Doppler tissue imaging; LA, left atrium; PW, pulse wave; DT, deceleration time. *Normal Doppler tissue imaging lateral e' ≥10 cm/s, septal e' ≥8 cm/s; ** left atrial volume ≥34 ml/m².

the synchronicity of contraction, improving left ventricular ejection fraction, reducing left ventricular volumes and increasing exercise tolerance.

There are two types of dyssynchrony:

1. Electrical dyssynchrony: these patients usually have broad left bundle branch block (LBBB) (QRS duration ≥150 ms), leading to delayed activation of the posterolateral wall compared to the septal wall.
2. Mechanical dyssynchrony may be present in the absence of electrical dyssynchrony (QRS <150 ms) due to impaired electromechanical coupling in diseased myocardium.

Dyssynchrony may be manifest at three different levels:

1. Interventricular: significant delay between left and right ventricular contraction.
2. Intraventricular: significant delay in contraction of different regions of the left ventricle.
3. Atrioventricular: abnormal timing of atrial and ventricular contraction results in suboptimal ventricular filling.

Echocardiographic assessment of ventricular dyssynchony

Severe dyssynchrony can often be appreciated on two-dimensional imaging as a rocking motion of the left ventricle (Fig. 5.6). More subtle dyssynchrony needs careful assessment, but at present there is no single definitive echocardiographic method for assessing dyssynchrony, nor any guarantee that the detection of dyssynchrony predicts a favourable response to CRT. The best evidence available from major clinical trials supports the use of DTI techniques.

Response rates to CRT appear to be highest in patients with intraventricular dyssynchrony with LBBB ≥150 ms: echocardiographic assessment of dyssynchrony

Figure 5.6

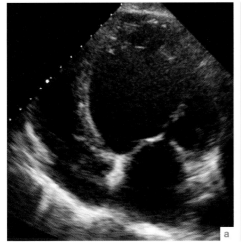

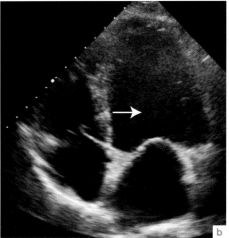

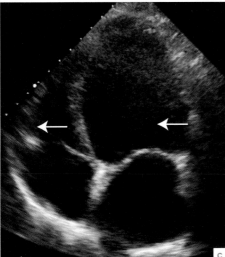

Obvious dyssynchrony. Apical four-chamber views. **(a)** End diastole. **(b)** Early systole is associated with septal contraction (arrow). **(c)** Late systole is associated with septal relaxation and simultaneous lateral wall contraction (arrows).

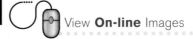

View **On-line** Images

Figure 5.7

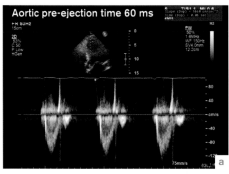
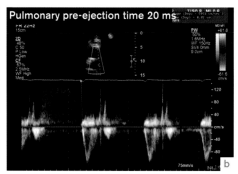

Assessment of interventricular dyssynchrony: pre-ejection times. (a) Pulse wave Doppler in left ventricular outflow tract. **(b)** Pulse wave Doppler in right ventricular outflow tract. Pre-ejection times are measured from the onset of the QRS to the beginning of forward flow on the Doppler spectra. A difference of 40 ms or more is considered significant.

in these patients is not required prior to CRT device implantation. However, echocardiographic assessment may be helpful in selecting patients with QRS <150 ms who may still benefit from CRT.

Interventricular dyssynchrony

Pre-ejection times

The overall timings of left and right ventricular contraction can be compared by analysing the delay between the onset of the QRS complex on the electrocardiograph and the onset of blood flow from left and right ventricles, respectively. This is known as the pre-ejection time, and is measured from standard PW Doppler recordings of blood flow in the left and right ventricular outflow tracts. A difference of more than 40 ms is considered significant (Fig. 5.7).

Intraventricular dyssynchrony

M-mode

Evidence of regional dyssynchrony within the left ventricle can be demonstrated using standard M-mode recordings from the parasternal long axis or mid ventricular parasternal short axis views to compare anteroseptal and posterior wall contraction. The time difference between the peak inward movement of the septal and posterior walls is measured. A difference of ≥130 ms between the two walls is indicative of significant intraventricular delay (Fig. 5.8).

This parameter is not considered definitive evidence of dyssynchrony for a variety of reasons. Firstly, septal movement can be complex, and it can be difficult to determine the point of peak movement. Secondly, it does not distinguish movement due to contraction from passive displacement.

Figure 5.8

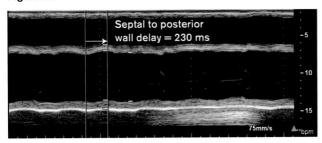

Septal to posterior wall delay = 230 ms

75mm/s

M-mode assessment of intraventricular dyssynchrony. Parasternal long axis view M-mode (sweep speed 75 mm/s). The delay between septal and posterior wall contraction is measured as shown. A delay of 130 ms or more is considered significant.

Figure 5.9

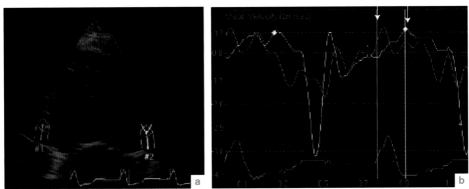

a

b

Colour-coded tissue Doppler analysis. (a) Colour TD two-dimensional image and sampling volumes at the septal and lateral walls are shown. **(b)** The velocity curves for each sample are displayed. Arrows indicate >100 ms delay between peak systolic tissue Doppler velocities of the septal and lateral walls.

Tissue Doppler imaging

Regional delays in left ventricular wall motion can be assessed much more accurately using Doppler tissue methods. The most reliable approach uses colour-coded DTI to compare the systolic velocities of opposing walls of the left ventricle (Fig. 5.9). Imaging is optimised in the A4C view to show the left ventricle and mitral annulus, and the colour DTI sector is set to cover the whole left ventricle with a high frame rate (>90 frames/s). Then 3–5 cardiac cycles are recorded for offline analysis. Potentially this can be repeated for each apical view so that all mid and basal segments can be analysed (i.e. 12 segments).

Sample volumes are positioned at symmetrical segments of opposing left ventricular walls (e.g. lateral and septal) and adjusted to give clear time–velocity spectra. Systolic velocities should only be measured during the left ventricular ejection period (from the beginning to the end of blood flow in the left ventricular outflow tract, as measured with pulse wave Doppler), and this can be superimposed on the time–velocity curve.

The time from QRS onset to peak systolic velocity is measured for each pair of opposing myocardial segments. The simplest approach is to compare two sites on opposing walls in the A4C view (e.g. basal lateral and septal velocities): a difference of 65 ms is considered significant. A more comprehensive analysis can involve up to 12 sites (mid and basal segments from the A4C, A2C and A3C views): a maximal difference of 100 ms or more or standard deviation ≥33 ms predicts response to CRT. There is little evidence to suggest that the more complex methods are any better than the simple two-site approach.

In reality most centres use real-time PW Doppler tissue imaging to measure the time from QRS onset to peak (or onset) systolic velocity at the lateral and septal walls of the mitral valve annulus from an A4C view (Fig. 5.10). The main

Figure 5.10

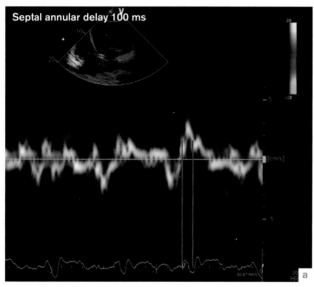

Pulse wave tissue Doppler assessment of intraventricular dyssynchrony. (a) Septal mitral annulus. **(b)** Lateral mitral annulus. Significant dyssynchrony between the medial and lateral left ventricular walls is evident.

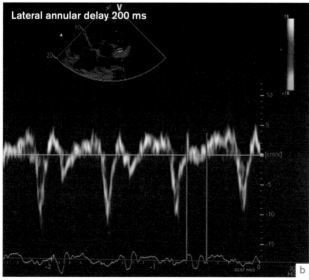

disadvantages of this method are the fact that it is less well validated, and different cardiac cycles are analysed for each site so there is more potential for error due to respiratory/patient movement.

Speckle tracking

Myocardium has a speckled appearance on standard two-dimensional grey-scale imaging, and software can be used to track the movement of these echodensities. This provides information about myocardial velocity and strain (percentage thickening). Segmental analysis of radial strain appears to hold promise as a method for detecting dyssynchrony (Fig. 5.11).

Real-time three-dimensional echo

Real-time three-dimensional echo can be used to assess regional dyssynchrony (see Chapter 21). The main advantage is the ability to analyse wall motion of all endocardial segments simultaneously during one cardiac cycle. However, the temporal resolution is relatively poor due to low frame rates. Schematic maps of segmental wall motion can be useful for localising and quantifying dyssynchrony (Fig. 5.12).

Figure 5.11

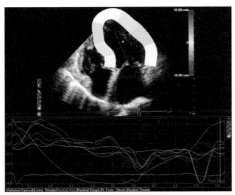

Speckle tracking. Apical four-chamber view. Colour-coded speckle tracking data is superimposed on a two-dimensional image of the left ventricle. In this example radial velocity is also displayed for each segment graphically in the bottom panel. No significant dyssynchrony is present.

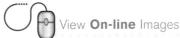 View **On-line** Images

Figure 5.12

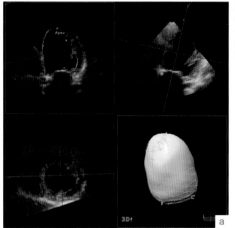

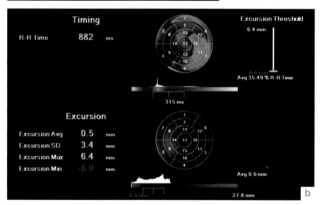

Real-time three-dimensional imaging. (a) Left ventricular endocardial border detection and three-dimensional reconstruction. **(b)** Segmental mapping of endocardial timing and excursion identifies areas of dyssynchrony.

CHAPTER

6

The right ventricle

The anatomy of the right ventricle

The right ventricle is very distinct from the left ventricle in many respects. It works at lower pressures than the left, and is therefore thinner-walled. In addition it is highly trabeculated and there is often a moderator band traversing the right ventricular cavity near the apex: this contains conducting tissue, and is entirely normal. Unlike the left ventricle, which has a relatively symmetrical shape, right ventricular geometry is complex and asymmetric: in cross-section it is crescentic, and it wraps around the left ventricle.

Blood flows in through the tricuspid valve, and exits via the right ventricular outflow tract (RVOT), which is essentially a funnel of muscle leading to the pulmonary valve.

Echocardiographic appearance

The entire right ventricle cannot be seen on any single echo view. It is best appreciated on the apical four-chamber (A4C) view, but is also seen on parasternal long axis (PSLAX), parasternal short axis (PSSAX), subcostal views, as well as the right ventricular inflow and outflow views of these positions (see Figs 2.5, 2.6, 2.8, 2.10 and 2.12).

The right ventricle should be thin-walled, and smaller than the left ventricle. Trabeculations usually appear as a velvety lining to the endocardium. The apex in the A4C view is narrow, and dominated by the left ventricular apex.

A moderator band often stretches from the interventricular septum to the right ventricular free wall near the apex. It is best seen in the A4C view (Fig. 6.1), and blends with the trabeculations of the right ventricle.

Figure 6.1

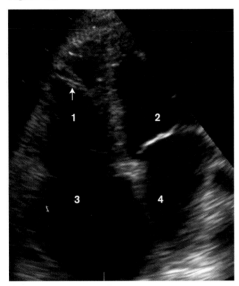

Moderator band. Apical four-chamber view. The moderator band is seen as a bundle of tissue in the apical right ventricle between the interventricular septum and right ventricular free wall (arrow).

1

2

3

4

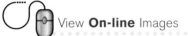
View **On-line** Images

Assessing the right ventricle

Structural assessment

The complex shape of the right ventricle makes structural assessment difficult. The overall size should be less than that of the left ventricle, and on the A4C view the left ventricle should form the apex of the heart. Significant right ventricular enlargement can lead to right ventricular dominance at the apex.

Standard linear measurements of the right ventricle are demonstrated in Figures 6.2 and 6.3. In the A4C view the diameter should be measured at the level of the tricuspid annulus (RVID1: normal ≤2.8 cm) and in the mid-ventricle (RVID2: normal ≤3.3 cm). Right ventricular length should be measured from the apex to the tricuspid annulus (RVID3: normal ≤7.9 cm). The mid right ventricular diameter can also be assessed in the PSLAX view, in the same manner described for the left ventricle (Fig. 6.2). Additional measurements include the RVOT diameter adjacent to the pulmonary valve (normal ≤2.3 cm) and aortic valves (normal ≤2.9 cm) in the PSSAX view (Fig. 6.3).

The thickness of the right ventricular free wall is best assessed on the subcostal view at the level of the tricuspid valve chordae. It should be less than 0.5 cm (Fig. 6.4).

Assessment of systolic function

Subjective and quantitative methods can be used to assess right ventricular function.

Figure 6.2

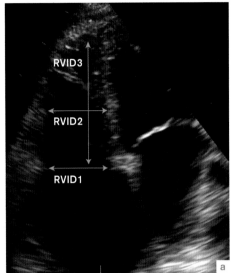

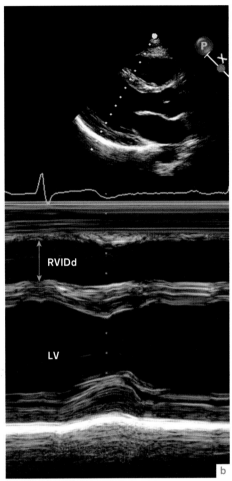

Right ventricular dimensions. (a) In the apical four-chamber view the following dimensions should be measured at end diastole: RVID1, basal right ventricular dimension at the level of the tricuspid annulus; RVID2, mid ventricular dimension; RVID3, right ventricular length from apex to base (mid-tricuspid annulus). **(b)** Parasternal long axis view M-mode. RVIDd, right ventricular diastolic internal diameter; LV, left ventricle.

Subjective assessment

It is difficult to assess right ventricular function because wall thickening is not easily appreciated, and the pattern of wall contraction is from both the apex and base towards the RVOT, which cannot be seen in a single view. An overall impression of right ventricular function can be made from observation of right ventricular movement in the A4C view. It is particularly helpful to concentrate on the movement of the tricuspid annulus towards the right ventricular apex.

Regional wall motion abnormalities may occur after myocardial infarction, but specific scoring systems are not in use.

Quantitative assessment

A variety of quantitative methods can be used in the A4C view:
1. Tricuspid annular plane systolic excursion (TAPSE): the M-mode beam is positioned through the lateral tricuspid annulus. Normal displacement

Figure 6.3

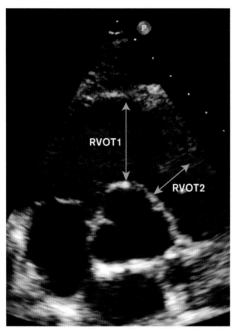

Right ventricular outflow tract (RVOT) dimensions. Parasternal short axis view at aortic valve level. RVOT1, Supra-aortic RVOT dimension at 12 o'clock position above aortic valve. RVOT2, Subpulmonic RVOT dimension at the pulmonary valve.

Figure 6.4

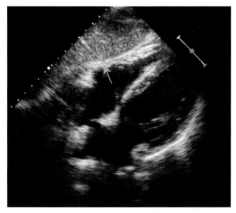

Measuring right ventricular free wall thickness. Subcostal view of the right ventricle: the free wall thickness is measured at the level of the tricuspid valve chordae at end diastole (arrows).

towards the apex is measured as shown in Figure 6.5 (normal 1.6–2.0 cm, mild 1.1–1.5 cm, moderate 0.6–1.0 cm, severe ≤0.5 cm).

2. Doppler tissue imaging: lateral tricuspid annual systolic velocity can be assessed on pulse wave Doppler tissue imaging. Normal peak systolic velocity is >10 cm/s.

3. Right ventricular fractional area change: the right ventricular endocardial border in the A4C view is traced in systole and diastole. The difference in right ventricular area reflects systolic function, but is not the same as ejection fraction. Normal is >30% (Fig. 6.6).

Figure 6.5

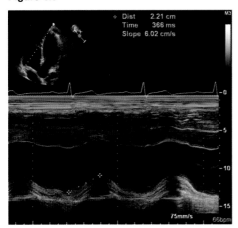

Tricuspid annular displacement. Tricuspid annular displacement towards the apex during systole can be measured using M-mode aligned with the lateral annulus.

Figure 6.6

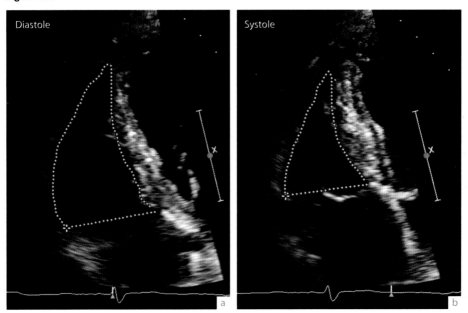

Right ventricular fractional area change. The right ventricular area is traced in systole and diastole from the apical four-chamber view. In this case there is a 52% change in area, suggesting normal right ventricular systolic function.

Assessment of diastolic function

In practice right ventricular diastolic function is rarely assessed. It can be categorised according to tricuspid inflow velocities on pulse wave Doppler (E:A ratio), analogous to the method already described for the left ventricle.

Normal E:A ratio is 1–1.5, impaired relaxation >1.5, pseudonormal 1–1.5 and restrictive >1.5. With abnormal diastolic function, blood flow patterns in the inferior vena cava/hepatic veins also become abnormal (diastolic dominant), and can be used to distinguish pseudonormal diastolic function from normal.

Reporting box

Reporting on the right ventricle

Summary

- Diagnosis
- Right ventricular structure and function
- Associated valvular disease
- Pulmonary hypertension

Qualitative data

- Structure of right ventricle: dilated, evidence of arrhythmogenic right ventricular cardiomyopathy
- Regional wall motion abnormalities
- Severity of associated valve lesions
- Evidence of intracardiac shunt, e.g. atrial septal defect, ventricular septal defect

Quantitative data

- Right ventricular dimensions
- Right ventricular fractional area change
- Right ventricular diastolic parameters
- Pulmonary artery pressure
- Pulmonary artery dimensions
- Right atrial dimensions
- Inferior vena cava dimensions
- Hepatic vein flow

The atria

Anatomy of the atria

The atria are the smallest cardiac chambers. They are roughly spherical and each has a small appendage located near the atrioventricular groove. The atria are separated by the interatrial septum, which contains the fossa ovalis. The right atrium receives blood from the inferior and superior vena cavae, and four pulmonary veins supply blood to the left atrium. Blood exits the atria via the atrioventricular valves to the respective ventricle.

The atria work at low pressure (5–10 mmHg) and are therefore thin-walled structures. At different stages of the cardiac cycle the atria work as pumps, reservoirs and conduits, thereby aiding ventricular filling.

Echocardiographic appearance

The left atrium is visible on many standard echocardiographic views, including parasternal long axis (PSLAX), parasternal short axis (PSSAX), apical, subcostal and even suprasternal views (Figs 2.5, 2.8, 2.10, 2.12 and 2.14). It is about half to a third of the size of a normal left ventricle. The left atrial appendage is not usually identifiable on transthoracic echocardiography, but can be readily visualised on transoesophageal echocardiography.

The interatrial wall is often poorly defined, partly because it is so thin in the region of the fossa ovalis, but also because it is usually parallel to the ultrasound beam, except in the subcostal view.

Four pulmonary veins insert into the posterior wall of the left atrium: some of these can be identified on the apical four-chamber (A4C) and suprasternal 'crab' view using colour flow mapping to demonstrate blood flow (Figs 2.14 and 13.11).

The right atrium is similar in size and shape to the left. It can be seen on the A4C, PSSAX and subcostal views (Figs 2.6, 2.8, 2.10 and 2.12). The connection of the inferior vena cava to the right atrium can be seen on the subcostal view: sometimes the superior vena cava can also be seen on a modified subcostal view.

Assessment of atrial structure

The left atrial anteroposterior diameter is routinely measured in atrial diastole from the PSLAX view using M-mode, or directly from the two-dimensional image (Fig. 7.1). As a rough estimate, this should be ≤4.0 cm. Atrial enlargement is often asymmetric, so it is better to estimate left atrial volume using the Simpson's biplane method. The geometry of the left atrium is defined in two planes by tracing the endocardial border in atrial diastole from the A4C and apical two-chamber (A2C) view (Fig. 7.2). Ideally this should be normalised to body surface area.

Figure 7.1

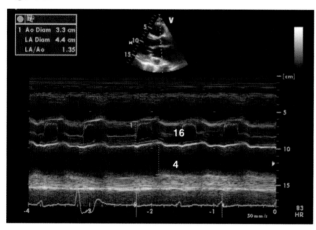

M-mode measurement of left atrial (LA) diameter. M-mode is aligned perpendicular to the aortic root on a parasternal long axis view. LA anteroposterior diameter is measured in atrial diastole.

Figure 7.2

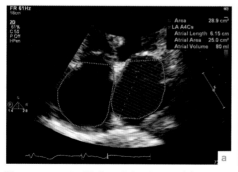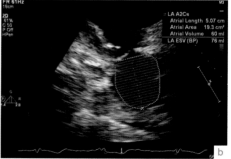

Measurement of left atrial volume. (a) Apical four-chamber view (A4C). **(b)** Apical two-chamber view (A2C). Left atrial geometry is defined by tracing the endocardial border in atrial diastole, in the A2C and A4C views. Right atrial area is also indicated.

Figure 7.3

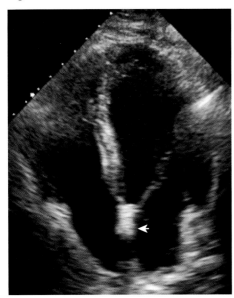

Lipomatous hypertrophy of the interatrial septum. Apical four-chamber view. The interatrial septum is generally thickened (arrowhead), with apparent dropout in the region of the fossa ovalis.

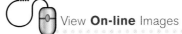
View **On-line** Images

The right atrium is not easily visible on two orthogonal views, so volume measurements are not possible. Instead, the diameter in the minor axis from the septal to lateral wall is measured from the A4C view (normal ≤4.5 cm). Alternatively, the right atrial area can be measured (Fig. 7.2).

Normal variants

Lipomatous hypertrophy of the interatrial septum

In this condition the interatrial septum is thickened, due to deposition of fatty material. It is not pathological and has no specific consequences. Thickening can be generalised or localised, but usually spares the fossa ovalis (Fig. 7.3). Localised thickening can be mistaken for tumour or thrombus.

Chiari network

The Chiari network is an embryological vestige that has a very ephemeral, wafting echocardiographic appearance. It is best seen on A4C and subcostal views (Fig. 7.4). Occasionally, objects such as thrombus get caught in the mesh of the network.

Eustachian valve

This is an endocardial ridge or fold that lies at the junction of the inferior vena cava and right atrium. It directs blood towards the fossa ovalis in the fetus, but

Figure 7.4

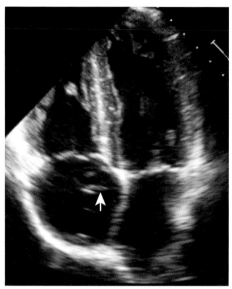

Chiari network. Apical four-chamber view. There is a prominent Chiari network in the right atrium (arrow). This is best appreciated on the video loop due to the characteristic wafting appearance. In addition, there is an atrial septal aneurysm.

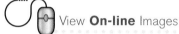
View **On-line** Images

Figure 7.5

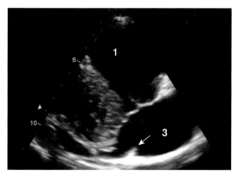

Eustachian valve. Parasternal long axis right ventricular inflow view. The eustachian valve (arrow) can be seen at the junction of the inferior vena cava and the right atrium. It directs blood flow towards the foramen ovale.

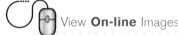
View **On-line** Images

has no significance in the adult. The commonest appearance is a small ridge, but it can be very elongated, and may be mistaken for thrombus or tumour. It can be seen in the A4C, subcostal and PSLAX right ventricular inflow views (Fig. 7.5).

Atrial diseases

Atrial enlargement

Atrial enlargement is very frequently detected as a consequence of other cardiac problems, particularly when ventricular filling pressures are raised (e.g. systolic or diastolic ventricular dysfunction), or if there is significant valvular disease (Fig. 7.6). In these situations atrial dilatation is often associated with atrial fibrillation

Figure 7.6

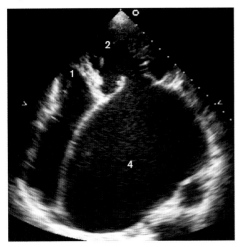

Left atrial enlargement. There is massive enlargement of the left atrium, which dwarfs the other chambers of the heart. The interatrial septum bulges towards the right ventricle, indicating raised left atrial pressure. The underlying cause is severe mitral regurgitation.

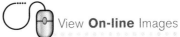
View **On-line** Images

Figure 7.7

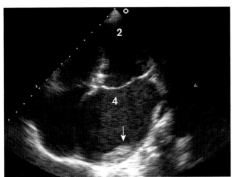

Spontaneous left atrial contrast and thrombus. Apical four-chamber view. This patient has severe rheumatic mitral valve disease, resulting in substantial left atrial enlargement. There is spontaneous echo contrast in the left atrium, seen swirling around on the video loop. A layer of thrombus is evident on the superior wall of the left atrium (arrow).

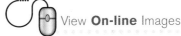
View **On-line** Images

due to disruption of normal electrical activity. Atrial dilatation may also occur as a result of chronic atrial fibrillation in the absence of other cardiac disease.

Spontaneous contrast and thrombus

Thrombus formation within the atria occurs most commonly in patients with atrial fibrillation. This is partly explained by stagnation of blood flow due to atrial dilatation and reduced atrial contractility. The risk of thrombosis is particularly high in rheumatic mitral valve disease, but many other conditions and factors can contribute to this as well. The major complication of left atrial thrombus is systemic embolisation, causing strokes, visceral infarcts and peripheral arterial emboli.

Around 90% of thrombi occur in the left atrial appendage, and can only be detected reliably by transoesophageal echo. However, large thrombi can occasionally be seen at other sites within the left atrium (Fig. 7.7).

Figure 7.8

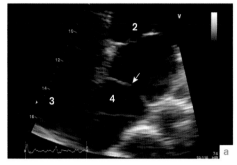

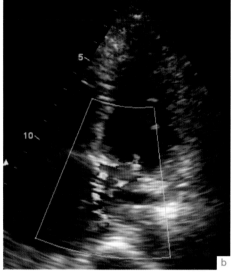

Cor triatriatum. Apical four-chamber view.
(a) There is a membrane subdividing the left atrium
(arrow). **(b)** Colour flow mapping demonstrates a
high-velocity jet passing through a small channel in
the membrane, along the interatrial septum and
towards the mitral valve.

View **On-line** Images

Spontaneous echo contrast is a description given to increased echogenicity within the blood pool, which has a swirling smoke-like appearance. This may represent microthrombi and is associated with increased risk of thrombosis.

Pulmonary emboli arise from peripheral venous thrombi. Very occasionally large emboli may be detected echocardiographically in the right atrium en route to the lungs.

Atrial masses

Atrial masses and tumours are considered in detail in Chapter 18.

Atrial septal defects

The classification and assessment of congenital atrial septal defects are covered in detail in Chapter 20.

Cor triatriatum

This is a congenital abnormality in which one of the atria is subdivided by an additional septum. The appearance is therefore of three atria, as the name suggests. The degree of obstruction to normal blood flow and associated congenital abnormalities determine the presentation: severe cases usually present at birth/ infancy with pulmonary oedema whereas milder cases can present in adulthood (Fig. 7.8).

Reporting box

Reporting on the atria

Summary

Comment on atrial size and any significant pathology

Qualitative

Atrial pathology/variants

- Thrombus
- Mass/tumour
- Eustachian valve
- Chiari network

Interatrial septal pathology/variants

- Patent foramen ovale
- Atrial septal aneurysm
- Atrial septal defect
- Lipomatous hypertrophy

Quantitative

Left atrial dimensions (indexed to body surface area)

- Anteroposterior dimension (M-mode)
- Biplane volume

Right atrial dimensions (indexed to body surface area)

- Dimensions in apical four-chamber view
- Area in apical four-chamber view
- Single plane area

Myocardial infarction

Introduction

Myocardial infarction (MI) is defined as death (necrosis) of myocardial tissue due to inadequate oxygen supply (ischaemia). The vast majority of MIs are caused by thrombotic occlusion of a coronary artery, usually precipitated by rupture of atherosclerotic plaque (Fig. 8.1). The consequences of this really depend on the site of the occlusion within the coronary anatomy, and whether or not blood flow is restored (reperfusion). In the worst-case scenario a major vessel occludes proximally, and the whole myocardial territory dies, which may trigger a cascade of immediate and long-term complications. At the other end of the scale a small side branch may occlude, with much less likelihood of complications.

Echocardiography is routinely undertaken in most patients following MI, principally to assess left ventricular function, but also to screen for other potential mechanical complications, which are discussed here.

Acute complications

Left ventricular dysfunction

Myocardial ischaemia/infarction immediately results in myocardial contractile dysfunction: echocardiographically this is manifest as a regional wall motion abnormality conforming to the affected coronary artery territory. The exact appearance depends on the site of thrombosis (proximal or distal vessel) and the collateral blood supply as well as individual anatomic variation.

Three coronary arteries supply distinct territories of myocardium that are relatively conserved between individuals

Figure 8.1

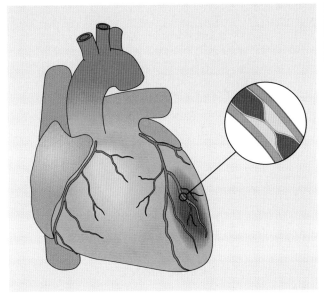

Pathophysiology of myocardial infarction.
Occlusion of a coronary artery results in a region of ischaemia/infarction in that territory.

Figure 8.2

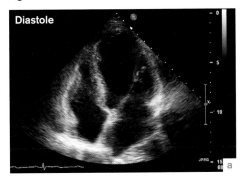

Diastole

Systole

a

b

Acute anterior myocardial infarction. Apical four-chamber view. **(a)** Diastole. **(b)** Systole. The left ventricle has normal wall thickness, but the anteroseptal region (arrows) fails to thicken in systole and is akinetic. All other areas thicken normally. This appearance is consistent with acute anteroseptal infarction due to occlusion of the left anterior descending artery in the mid vessel.

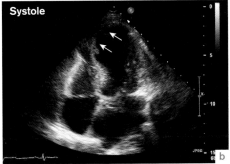 View On-line Images

(Fig. 4.7). Occlusion of the left anterior descending artery therefore causes anterior wall motion abnormalities (Fig. 8.2). Likewise, occlusion of the right coronary artery causes inferior regional wall motion abnormalities (Fig. 10.1).

In the setting of acute MI, it is not possible to be sure whether an otherwise normal-appearing akinetic segment represents an area of irreversible infarction, or if the myocardium is stunned and temporarily dysfunctional. Restoration of blood flow may salvage viable myocardium, and functional recovery may ensue over days or weeks. In contrast, thinned, echo-bright, akinetic myocardium represents prior (weeks–years) myocardial injury (see Fig. 8.8, below).

Right ventricular dysfunction

Right ventricular infarction occurs in around 50% of all inferior MIs, and is clinically apparent in about 10%. It is usually due to proximal occlusion of the right coronary artery, leading to acute right ventricular failure and cardiogenic shock.

Acute echo features of right ventricular infarction include right ventricular dilatation, systolic impairment, regional wall motion abnormality, paradoxical septal motion and acute tricuspid regurgitation (Fig. 10.1). In the long term, echocardiographic evidence of scarring and remodelling may become apparent.

Myocardial rupture

Acutely infarcted myocardium is structurally weak and prone to spontaneous rupture: fortunately this is quite rare. The exact consequences and echocardiographic appearance depend on the site of rupture.

Ventricular free wall rupture

Ventricular free wall rupture causes catastrophic leakage of blood at high pressure into the pericardial space, leading to cardiac tamponade (Fig. 8.3). It is invariably fatal, and accounts for around 10% of all in-hospital deaths from acute MI.

A partial rupture may lead to pseudoaneurysm formation, in which pericardial haematoma prevents further blood leak. The haematoma can be mistaken for aneurysmal myocardium; however, unlike a true aneurysm, the neck is narrow, representing the site of rupture (Fig. 8.4). Surgical repair of a pseudoaneurysm rupture may be feasible.

Figure 8.3

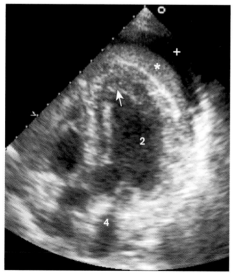

Ventricular free wall rupture. Apical four-chamber view. There is pericardial haematoma (*) and an echo-free space (+), which probably represents fresh blood leak. In addition there is evidence of discontinuity in the left ventricular wall at the apex (arrow), suggesting this is the site of rupture. The left atrium is compressed. Overall the appearances suggest that this patient developed a pseudoaneurysm which eventually leaked, causing acute tamponade.

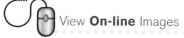 View **On-line** Images

Ventricular septal rupture

Haemorrhage into a septal infarct can lead to rupture and the formation of a ventricular septal defect. This results in shunting of blood from the left ventricle to the right ventricle, often causing haemodynamic collapse and cardiogenic shock. Emergency surgical repair of the defect is indicated.

The myocardium adjacent to an ischaemic ventricular septal defect is often abnormally thickened due to tissue swelling and oedema. Blood flow across the defect is usually apparent on colour flow mapping (Fig. 8.5). Standard views may miss a ventricular septal defect, and if the diagnosis is strongly suspected on clinical grounds, the septum should be scrutinised from as many views as possible.

Papillary muscle rupture: acute mitral regurgitation

The mitral valve is particularly susceptible to myocardial dysfunction because of the importance of normal papillary muscle function for valve integrity. Acute mitral regurgitation in the context of an acute MI is usually due to papillary muscle ischaemia. This is more common with inferoposterior infarction affecting the posteromedial papillary muscle group since it has a single arterial blood supply. The infarct territory is often quite small.

Ischaemia causes impaired papillary muscle relaxation, which restricts movement of the posterior mitral valve leaflet and leads to failure of coaptation with

Figure 8.4

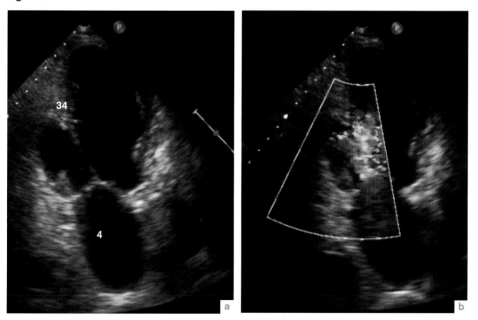

Pseudoaneurysm. Apical three-chamber view. **(a)** A pseudoaneurysm is present in the inferior left ventricular wall. This has a characteristic rim of myocardium at the neck of the aneurysm, and the pericardial space is filled with thrombus. **(b)** Colour flow mapping demonstrates blood flow into the pseudoaneurysm.

View **On-line** Images

Figure 8.5

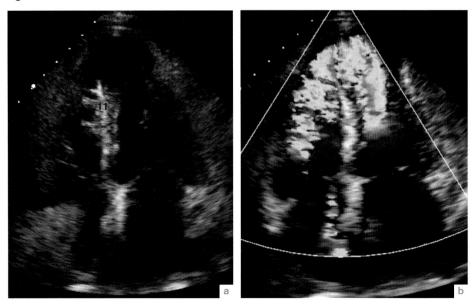

Ventricular septal rupture. A4C views. **(a)** There is a large break in the interventricular septum at the apex. **(b)** Colour flow mapping demonstrates turbulent blood flow from the left to the right ventricle.

View **On-line** Images

the tip of the anterior leaflet. Papillary function will often improve with successful reperfusion, leading to resolution of mitral regurgitation. Papillary muscle ischaemia can be inferred if there is posterior or inferior akinesis, with an eccentric mitral regurgitant jet, and intact papillary muscles. Movement of the posterior mitral leaflet may appear restricted. The regurgitant jet is usually directed posteriorly, towards the abnormal leaflet: this is in contrast to the situation in mitral valve prolapse where the regurgitant jet is directed away from the prolapsing leaflet.

Less frequently, acute mitral regurgitation may be caused by complete or partial rupture of a papillary muscle, secondary to infarction (Fig. 8.6). This leads to catastrophic mitral regurgitation and acute pulmonary oedema, which is often fatal. Emergency surgical repair or replacement of the mitral valve is indicated.

Papillary muscle rupture may be directly visualised on transthoracic echocardiography and appears as a stump or free portion attached to the mitral valve leaflet or papillary base. Alternatively, rupture may be inferred from demonstrating a flail mitral leaflet/segment. Transoesophageal echocardiography will identify the exact pathology more reliably.

Standard echo measures underestimate the severity of acute mitral regurgitation, largely because acute elevation of left atrial pressure reduces the apparent size of the mitral regurgitation jet on colour flow mapping Doppler. The most reliable parameter in this situation is the vena contracta width. A diagnostic clue that mitral regurgitation may be more severe than initially perceived is that left ventricular function often appears to be paradoxically good despite clinical evidence of cardiogenic shock.

Figure 8.6

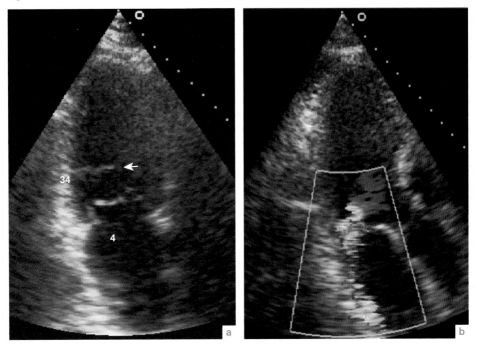

Acute mitral regurgitation. (a) Apical two-chamber view. **(b)** Apical three-chamber view. One head of the posteromedial papillary muscle group is disconnected from the mitral valve leaflets (arrow). This causes a posteriorly directed eccentric jet of mitral regurgitation, consistent with excessive anterior mitral valve leaflet movement.

View **On-line** Images

Mural thrombus

Thrombus formation occurs due to endocardial damage and stagnation of blood adjacent to akinetic infarcted myocardium. Thrombus characteristically appears homogeneous, and may be globular/pedunculated and mobile, or laminated and static (Fig. 8.7). Detection requires a high degree of suspicion because it can easily be missed, either because it is small and hidden on some views, or because it resembles normal myocardium. In the absence of a significant wall motion abnormality, the likelihood of thrombus is low. Mural thrombus is discussed more in Chapter 18.

Pericarditis

Acute pericarditis post acute MI is common and usually self-limiting. It represents transmural infarction causing epicardial/pericardial inflammation. The effusion is usually small and virtually undetectable on echo, and has no particular distinguishing features. MI can trigger an autoimmune reaction that results in recurrent episodes of pericarditis weeks later. This is known as Dressler's syndrome. Again, there are no particular distinguishing echocardiographic features.

Figure 8.7

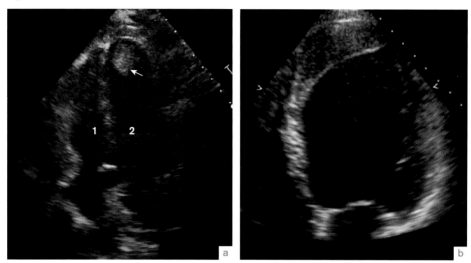

Mural thrombus. **(a)** The apex of the left ventricle is filled with mobile thrombus (arrow) following an anterior myocardial infarct a few days earlier. **(b)** Chronic laminated apical thrombus.

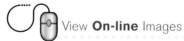

View **On-line** Images

Figure 8.8

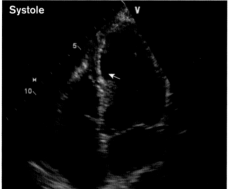

Myocardial scar. Apical four-chamber view. The anteroseptal wall is echo-bright, and akinetic (arrow). This represents an area of chronic scarring.

View **On-line** Images

Chronic complications

Left ventricular remodelling

Remodelling describes the left ventricular structural changes that occur following acute MI. Infarcted tissue is replaced by scar over a period of weeks to months, and may be associated with left ventricular dilatation, systolic/diastolic dysfunction and compensatory hypertrophy of non-infarcted segments. Frequently this is associated with clinical signs of heart failure.

Echocardiographically, scar appears as thinned akinetic/dyskinetic myocardium, with increased echogenicity (Fig. 8.8). Aneurysm formation occurs when weak scar

Figure 8.9

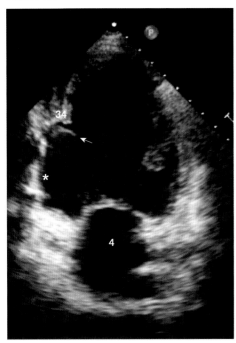

Inferior wall aneurysm. Apical two-chamber view. A true aneurysm (*) can be seen in the basal/mid segments of the inferior left ventricular wall. Thrombus is present within the aneurysm (arrow).

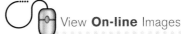
View **On-line** Images

tissue expands outwards, forming an abnormal dilatation in the ventricular wall. Aneurysms appear as a region of bulging, thinned, hyperreflectant ventricular tissue, connected to the rest of the left ventricle by a wide neck (Fig. 8.9). They display evidence of dyskinesis (paradoxical outward movement), but this is often difficult to demonstrate unequivocally on echo. Apical aneurysms are most common, but they can occur in any location.

Chronic mitral regurgitation

Mitral regurgitation in the chronic phase after MI usually occurs as a result of disruption of the subvalvular apparatus due to left ventricular remodelling. Significant ventricular dilatation can displace the papillary muscles and stretch the subvalvular apparatus so that proper leaflet coaptation cannot occur. In addition, left ventricular dilatation can be associated with mitral annular dilatation, which in itself can disrupt normal valve closure. Such changes generally occur in the presence of severe left ventricular dysfunction, and the mitral regurgitant jet is centrally directed (Fig. 8.10). Significant functional mitral regurgitation can add to the volume burden of the left ventricle, precipitating a vicious cycle of declining left ventricular function and worsening mitral regurgitation. In general this mechanism is not amenable to surgical repair or valve replacement.

Another potential mechanism is papillary muscle infarction and scarring, which lead to papillary shortening and retraction of one or other mitral leaflet. This process usually affects the posteromedial papillary group. In general the

Figure 8.10

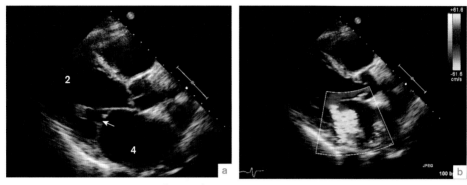

Functional mitral regurgitation. (a and **b)** Parasternal long axis views. There is significant left ventricular dilatation following previous myocardial infarction. There is failure of leaflet tip coaptation (arrow) leading to functional mitral regurgitation.

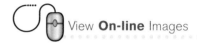 View **On-line** Images

Figure 8.11

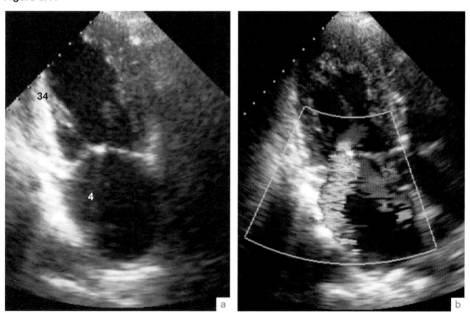

Chronic papillary muscle dysfunction. (a) Apical two-chamber view. **(b)** Apical three-chamber view. The inferior wall and papillary muscle are akinetic and echo-bright, suggesting fibrosis. The eccentric jet of mitral regurgitation is directed posteriorly, suggesting that posterior mitral valve leaflet closure is restricted.

(page View **On-line** Images

echocardiographic appearance is of a posteroinferior wall motion abnormality, with restricted posterior leaflet movement and an eccentric, posteriorly directed mitral regurgitant jet (Fig. 8.11). Left ventricular function is often quite good. Severe regurgitation in this situation may be amenable to mitral valve repair.

Reporting box

Reporting on myocardial infarction

Summary

- Comment on global left and right ventricular systolic function
- Comment on major complications

Qualitative data

- Regional wall motion abnormalities
- Regions of scar, aneurysm, hypertrophy
- Thrombus
- Ventricular septal defect, pseudoaneurysm, papillary rupture
- Pericardial effusion

Quantitative data

- Left ventricle: dimensions, fractional shortening, volumes, ejection fraction, left ventricular mass, E:A ratio, deceleration time, E;e' ratio
- Right ventricle: dimensions, fractional area change, tricuspid annular plane systolic excursion (TAPSE)

The cardiomyopathies

Cardiomyopathy is a rather non-specific term used to indicate disease of cardiac muscle, usually of unknown cause. There are three main types, classified according to left ventricular pathophysiology: namely, hypertrophic, dilated and restrictive cardiomyopathy.

Hypertrophic cardiomyopathy

Hypertrophic cardiomyopathy (HCM) is a genetic condition in which severe left ventricular thickening (hypertrophy) occurs in the absence of an identifiable secondary cause such as hypertension. When there is evidence of obstruction to blood flow in the ventricle or left ventricular outflow tract (LVOT), the condition is termed hypertrophic obstructive cardiomyopathy (HOCM). The majority of cases involve mutation of genes encoding sarcomeric proteins, but it is not currently understood how this causes the cardiac phenotype. The clinical manifestations vary substantially in severity and timing of onset between patients and families.

The echocardiographic features of HCM include the following:

1. **Left ventricular hypertrophy (LVH)** is the cardinal feature of HCM. The commonest pattern is asymmetric septal hypertrophy (ASH) (Fig. 9.1), in which the interventricular septal thickness is usually 15 mm or more, and the ratio of interventricular septal thickness to posterior wall thickness on M-mode is ≥1.3:1. Less common patterns of HCM include isolated hypertrophy of the left ventricular free wall, apical hypertrophy (Fig. 9.2) or concentric LVH. Usually the left ventricular cavity is small, and hypertrophy may be so severe as to cause almost complete obliteration of the cavity during systole (Fig. 9.1).

Cavity dimensions and wall thickness need to be carefully assessed due to the complex patterns of hypertrophy. Start with M-mode measurements from the parasternal long axis (PSLAX) view to determine interventricular septal and posterior wall thickness. Then measure wall thickness in quadrants from parasternal short axis (PSSAX) views (Fig. 9.3) at the basal (mitral), mid (papillary) and apical levels. Take care to avoid off-axis measurements and papillary muscles. Finally, assess left ventricular volumes (and ejection fraction) using Simpson's biplane method from apical views.

2. **Right ventricular hypertrophy** (>0.5 cm) often occurs in combination with LVH. Assess right ventricular free wall thickness in the PSSAX, subcostal and apical four-chamber views.

3. **Systolic anterior motion (SAM)** of the mitral valve is a term used to describe abnormal movement of the anterior mitral valve leaflet towards the interventricular septum (IVS) during systole. This is thought to be due to a suction force (Venturi effect) created as blood accelerates past the obstructing IVS, but other factors, such as abnormal mitral valve leaflets or papillary muscle positions, probably also contribute. SAM is best appreciated on PSLAX mitral valve M-mode recordings, and can be very difficult to detect on real-time two-dimensional images (Fig. 9.1).

4. **LVOT obstruction** can occur as a consequence of both severe septal thickening and SAM. Obstruction is characteristically dynamic, in that it gets progressively worse throughout systole, unlike aortic stenosis, which is a fixed obstruction that does not vary during the cardiac cycle. The continuous wave (CW) Doppler spectrum through the LVOT/aortic valve is often characteristically scimitar-shaped, with a late peak velocity (Fig. 9.1d and Fig. 9.4), reflecting increased obstruction as systole progresses. CW Doppler is useful in obtaining an accurate value for the gradient, but does not provide information about the location of the obstruction. This may be obvious if there is clear evidence of SAM and septal hypertrophy, but sometimes obstruction actually occurs at other sites in the left ventricular cavity due to septal hypertrophy. This can be confirmed by 'mapping' the pressure gradient within the left ventricular cavity, LVOT and aorta using pulse wave Doppler at each site (Fig. 9.4). A severe intracavitary gradient may reduce pressure in the LVOT sufficiently to allow aortic valve closure during late systole (premature aortic valve closure). This can be assessed on M-mode recordings (Fig. 9.1f). More commonly, the aortic valve cusps flutter due to turbulent blood flow.

The pressure gradient may not be evident at rest but can be provoked by manoeuvres that increase contractility or reduce preload/afterload, such as exercise, nitrate or dobutamine infusion.

5. **Diastolic dysfunction**: the degree of diastolic dysfunction is very variable and unrelated to the degree of hypertrophy. High left ventricular filling pressures caused by diastolic dysfunction can lead to atrial dilatation, and atrial fibrillation.

6. **Mitral regurgitation** can occur as a consequence of SAM, as well as mitral leaflet elongation and abnormal papillary muscle attachments. As the mitral

Figure 9.1

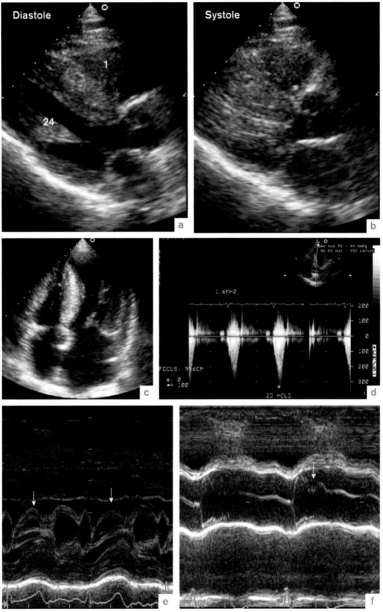

Hypertrophic obstructive cardiomyopathy. (a and **b)** Parasternal long axis view. **(c)** Apical four-chamber view. **(d)** Left ventricular outflow tract continuous wave Doppler. **(e)** Mitral valve M-mode. **(f)** Aortic valve M-mode. **(a–c)** Evidence of severe asymmetric septal hypertrophy can be seen in all views, with virtual obliteration of the left ventricular cavity in systole. **(d)** Continuous wave Doppler demonstrates a left ventricular outflow tract gradient of 44 mmHg at rest. The contour of the Doppler spectrum is scimitar-shaped, in keeping with a dynamic obstruction. **(e)** Systolic anterior motion of the anterior mitral valve leaflet can be seen on M-mode (arrows). This appears as a displacement of the leaflet towards the septum in late systole. **(f)** Premature closure of the aortic valve during mid-systole (arrow).

View **On-line** Images

Figure 9.2

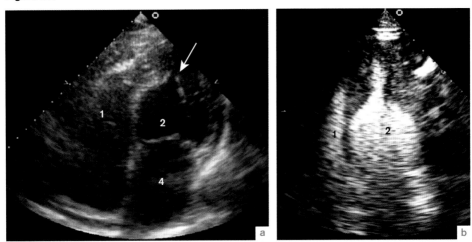

Apical hypertrophic cardiomyopathy. (a) Apical four-chamber (A4C) view. **(b)** A4C view using left ventricular contrast agent. There is a characteristic 'ace of spades' appearance. In systole the apex is obliterated (arrow).

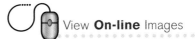 View **On-line** Images

Figure 9.3

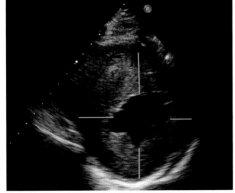

Segmental assessment of wall thickness. Parasternal short axis view: mid left ventricular level. Measure wall thickness in quadrants as shown, in the apical, papillary and mitral valve views.

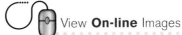 View **On-line** Images

valve is sucked towards the septum it becomes incompetent, causing mid/late systolic mitral regurgitation.

7. **Dilated cardiomyopathy:** HCM can 'burn out', leading to progressive wall thinning and ventricular dilatation with systolic dysfunction.

ASH, SAM and dynamic LVOT obstruction are not unique to HCM and the detection of these abnormalities needs to be considered in the context of the clinical situation (Table 9.1).

Complications of HCM include symptoms of angina, heart failure, syncope, sudden death, heart failure, atrial fibrillation, mitral regurgitation and infective

Figure 9.4

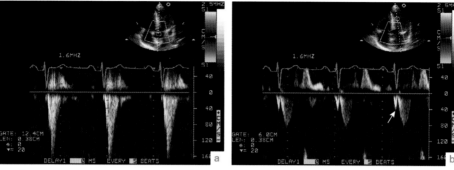

Localisation of outflow tract gradient. (a) Pulse wave Doppler sampling localised at the aortic valve gives a peak velocity in excess of 1.6 m/s. **(b)** Sampling in the left ventricular cavity gives a peak velocity of only 0.8 m/s. Acceleration of blood between the left ventricular cavity and aortic valve suggests the presence of mild left ventricular outflow tract obstruction. Further sampling points can be used to define the region of obstruction more precisely. The arrow indicates presystolic forward flow, which is sometimes seen in hypertrophic cardiomyopathy. This represents flow caused by atrial contraction against the stiff left ventricle.

Table 9.1 Alternative causes of ASH, SAM and LVOT obstruction

	Cause
ASH	Hypertensive LVH
	Posterior myocardial infarction
SAM	Hypercontractile states (e.g. during DSE, hypovolaemia, septic shock)
	Mitral valve repair
	Congenital papillary muscle abnormalities
	Acute myocardial infarction
	Transposition of the great arteries
LVOT obstruction	Severe hypertensive LVH (during DSE)
	Congenital papillary muscle abnormalities
	Acute myocardial infarction
	Takotsubo cardiomyopathy

ASH, asymmetric septal hypertrophy; SAM, systolic anterior motion of the mitral valve; LVOT, left ventricular outflow tract; LVH, left ventricular hypertrophy; DSE, dobutamine stress echo.

Figure 9.5

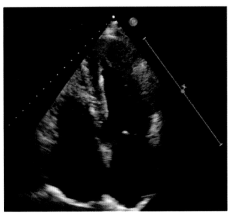

Anderson–Fabry cardiomyopathy. Apical four-chamber view. Note the bright endocardial septal border and apical hypertrophy.

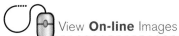
View **On-line** Images

endocarditis. Prognosis is dependent on the risk of sudden cardiac death due to ventricular arrhythmias. This correlates with very severe hypertrophy (IVS thickness >30 mm). Surprisingly, the severity of outflow tract obstruction on echo is a weak predictor of outcome.

Anderson–Fabry disease

This is an inherited disorder of metabolism (α-galactosidase deficiency) which can result in LVH similar to HCM. The echocardiographic appearance overlaps with that of HCM. Sometimes there is a distinct bright endocardial layer (Fig. 9.5), though this is by no means specific for this condition.

Athlete's heart

High-level training for endurance sports such as rowing, swimming and triathlons can cause eccentric cardiac hypertrophy due to volume loading of the left ventricle. This is considered physiological, reversible and benign. Sports such as weight lifting impose a pressure load on the heart and lead to concentric LVH. This pattern of hypertrophy may not be so benign.

Occasional difficulty arises in distinguishing between HCM and athlete's heart. Various criteria can be used to try to differentiate, though it is not an exact science (Table 9.2).

Dilated cardiomyopathy

Dilated cardiomyopathy is the end stage of many disparate cardiac pathologies that result in irreversible myocardial damage (Table 9.3): frequently an underlying cause cannot be identified. It is characterised by left ventricular dilatation, global

Table 9.2 Features distinguishing hypertrophic cardiomyopathy (HCM) and athlete's heart

Characteristic	Athlete's heart	HCM
Background	Elite endurance athletes	Family history of HCM
Training effect	Regression with abstinence	No regression
Dimensions	Diastolic interventricular septal thickness <1.6 cm	No limit
	Diastolic left ventricular internal diameter >55 mm	<45 mm
Systolic function	Normal	May be abnormal
Diastolic function	Normal/improved	Abnormal

Table 9.3 Common causes of dilated cardiomyopathy

Cause

Idiopathic (i.e. no cause identified)

Ischaemic heart disease

Valvular heart disease

Hypertension

Alcohol abuse

Viral myocarditis

Familial cardiomyopathy

Chemotherapy (anthracyclines, Herceptin)

hypokinesia and thinned left ventricular walls (Fig. 9.6). Echo examination should include assessment of left ventricular systolic and diastolic function, a possible underlying cause, secondary complications (e.g. functional mitral regurgitation) and evidence of left ventricular mechanical dyssynchrony.

Assessment of the underlying cause

In general it is not possible to determine the cause of a dilated cardiomyopathy from an echo study, and the medical history of the patient is most informative (e.g.

Figure 9.6

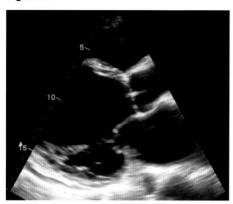

Dilated cardiomyopathy. Parasternal long axis view. The left ventricle is dilated (diastolic left ventricular internal diameter 7.5 cm) and globally hypocontractile, with very little evidence of left ventricular wall thickening or movement in systole.

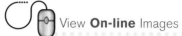

View **On-line** Images

history of prior myocardial infarction, family history of cardiomyopathy, alcohol abuse). However there may be specific clues, so it is important to look for evidence of severe valvular disease, LVH (suggesting hypertensive heart disease or HCM) or regional wall motion abnormalities (suggesting underlying ischaemic heart disease). Some cardiomyopathies have distinctive echocardiographic appearances that are discussed below.

Left ventricular non-compaction (LVNC)

This cardiomyopathy has a very distinctive appearance, characterised by the presence of discrete layers of normal (compact) and spongy (non-compact) myocardium at the apex/lateral free wall (Fig. 9.7a). Often, blood flow within small cavities in the spongy layer can be demonstrated on colour flow mapping Doppler. The spectrum of LVNC may also include a meshwork of trabeculations (Fig. 9.7b), or multiple prominent trabeculations, with deep blood-filled recesses (Fig. 9.7c and d). Unfortunately, there is no consensus definition, and it is well recognised that prominent trabeculations can be seen in normal people who do not have a cardiomyopathy. Sometimes apical HCM, mural thrombus and foreshortened apical views can give similar appearances.

LVNC generally presents in childhood/early adulthood and sometimes there is an underlying genetic predisposition. It may be associated with congenital heart defects and is believed to be a developmental disorder. As with all dilated cardiomyopathies, there is an increased risk of sudden cardiac death, arrhythmias and cardiac emboli.

Takotsubo cardiomyopathy

This is a distinct cardiomyopathy that often presents in a manner similar to an acute myocardial infarct, except that there is no evidence of significant coronary

Figure 9.7

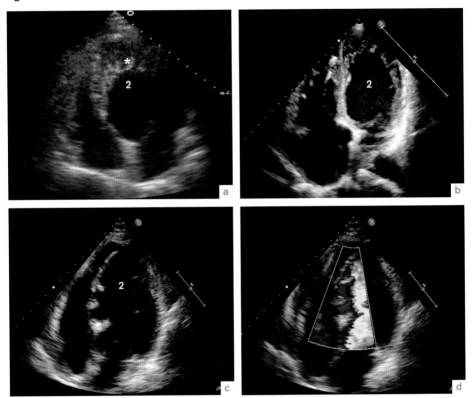

Isolated ventricular non-compaction. Apical four-chamber views. **(a)** Characteristic spongy appearance of the endocardial layer (*), with a more normal epicardial layer. **(b)** Trabecular meshwork pattern. **(c)** Multiple large trabeculations are present within the septal myocardium. **(d)** Blood flow in the recesses between trabeculations is clearly seen.

View **On-line** Images

artery disease. Typically, patients are acutely unwell with chest pain, electrocardiographic changes suggesting infarction, and signs of heart failure/cardiogenic shock. The name is Japanese for 'octopus pot' due to the appearance of the left ventricle on ventriculography (Fig. 9.8). Frequently the event is triggered by an extreme emotional shock, and for this reason it is sometimes referred to as 'broken heart' syndrome. The aetiology is thought to be mediated by profound release of adrenaline and related compounds from sympathetic nerves supplying the heart. In the majority of patients left ventricular function returns to normal over a period of weeks.

Echocardiography shows extensive akinesis of most of the left ventricle with hyperdynamic basal segments (Fig. 9.8). Occasionally the highly abnormal pattern of contraction leads to SAM of the mitral valve, causing dynamic left ventricular outflow obstruction and mitral regurgitation.

Figure 9.8

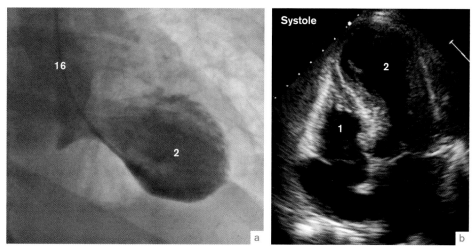

Takotsubo cardiomyopathy. (a) Left ventriculogram: characteristic 'octopus pot' appearance on ventriculography. The left ventricle is opacified with X-ray contrast medium, injected through a catheter. During systole only the basal segments contract, whilst the rest of the ventricle balloons outwards. **(b)** Apical four-chamber view, systole: the mid and apical segments are akinetic.

View **On-line** Images

Assessment of left ventricular function

This topic is covered in detail in Chapters 4 and 5, but a few points merit specific mention here. Accurate quantitative assessment of left ventricular function is essential as it is the most important prognostic indicator available, as well as determining eligibility for certain therapies, such as implantable cardioverter defibrillators and cardiac resynchronisation therapy.

Basic information about left ventricular systolic function should include measurement of left ventricular dimensions and biplane estimation of ejection fraction. Diastolic function is also important because patients with restrictive physiology have a poorer prognosis than those with lesser degrees of diastolic dysfunction.

Restrictive cardiomyopathy

Restrictive cardiomyopathy is characterised by extreme ventricular stiffness, which leads to severe diastolic dysfunction. It is caused by a wide range of conditions, most notably cardiac amyloidosis. This is associated with deposition of abnormal proteins or fibrosis in the myocardium, which leads to LVH and abnormal myocardial distensibility. The back-pressure caused by impaired left ventricular filling leads to gross atrial enlargement.

Figure 9.9

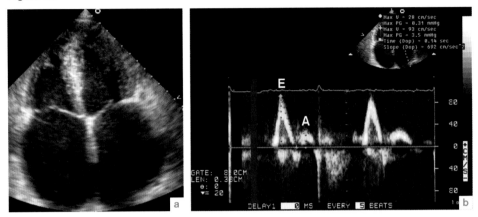

Restrictive cardiomyopathy. (a) Apical four-chamber view. **(b)** Mitral inflow pulse wave Doppler. There is severe left and right ventricular hypertrophy and severe biatrial enlargement. Mitral valve inflow pulse wave Doppler suggests restrictive diastolic physiology with E:A ratio of approximately 3:1 and deceleration time 140 ms. The speckling of the septum suggests an underlying diagnosis of amyloidosis.

View **On-line** Images

Echocardiographic features usually include marked biventricular hypertrophy, biatrial dilatation, near-normal left ventricular systolic function and restrictive diastolic physiology (E:A wave ratio ≤ 2, E wave deceleration time « 160 ms), with markedly elevated left ventricular filling pressure (E/e' ratio ≥ 13) (Fig. 9.9). Amyloidosis can cause a characteristic speckled myocardial texture, particularly in the septum, and valvular thickening.

Constrictive pericarditis can cause a similar clinical picture of biatrial enlargement with diastolic filling abnormalities. Although the echocardiographic features are often distinct, there is significant overlap and other imaging modalities may be required to reach a firm diagnosis.

Endomyocardial fibrosis

This is a specific form of restrictive cardiomyopathy characterised by the formation of endocardial scar tissue. Typically there is obliteration of one or both ventricular apices, but fibrosis of other areas can also occur. It is common in the tropics, but rare in developed countries. The underlying cause is not known.

On echo the ventricular volumes are reduced due to thick echo-bright material filling the apices, sometimes with overlying thrombus (Fig. 9.10). The atria are often dilated.

Figure 9.10

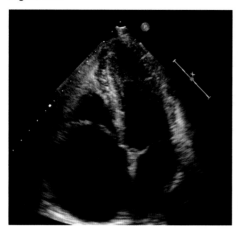

Endomyocardial fibrosis. Both ventricular apices are filled by fibrotic tissue, causing reduced cavity size: systolic function is preserved. The atria are severely dilated.

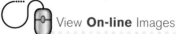
View **On-line** Images

Reporting box

Reporting on hypertrophic cardiomyopathy

Summary

- Diagnosis: hypertrophic cardiomyopathy
- Severity of hypertrophy
- Functional effect: outflow obstruction, systolic/diastolic function
- Complications, e.g. mitral regurgitation

Qualitative data

- Pattern of hypertrophy: asymmetric, concentric, apical, etc.
- Systolic anterior motion of the mitral valve: severity
- Premature aortic valve closure
- Localisation of obstruction: outflow, mid-cavity
- Evidence of complications

Quantitative data

- Left ventricular dimensions and wall thickness
  - Parasternal long axis M-mode dimensions
  - Parasternal short axis (PSSAX) basal, mid and apical wall thicknesses
- Right ventricular wall thickness
  - PSSAX, subcostal, apical four-chamber
- Left atrial volume
- Left ventricular volumes and ejection fraction
- Diastolic parameters: E:A ratio, deceleration time, E:e' ratio
- Left ventricular outflow tract gradient

Reporting box

Reporting on dilated cardiomyopathy

Summary

- Grade of global systolic and diastolic left ventricular (LV) function
- Right ventricular (RV) structure and function
- Severity of dilatation
- Comment on complications

Qualitative data

- Regional wall motion abnormalities
- Regions of scar, aneurysm, hypertrophy
- Complications: mitral regurgitation, thrombus, etc.

Quantitative data

- LV dimensions
- LV volumes
- LV mass
- Ejection fraction
- Fractional shortening
- Wall motion score index
- Diastolic parameters: E:A ratio, deceleration time, E;e' ratio
- RV dimensions
- RV fractional area change
- Pulmonary artery pressure

Reporting box

Reporting on restrictive cardiomyopathy

Summary

- Diagnosis
- Evidence of underlying aetiology (e.g. amyloid, endomyocardial fibrosis)
- Severity of hypertrophy
- Severity of systolic and diastolic dysfunction

Qualitative data

- Interpretation of diastolic parameters
- Pulmonary and hepatic vein flow pattern

Quantitative data

- Left ventricular (LV) dimensions
- LV mass
- LV ejection fraction and fractional shortening
- Tissue Doppler velocities
- Diastolic parameters: peak E wave velocity, E:A ratio, reversibility, E:e' ratio
- Inferior vena cava diameter
- Pulmonary artery pressure
- Atrial dimensions

CHAPTER

10

Right ventricular pathologies

A variety of pathologies can predominantly affect the right ventricular myocardium, and merit discussion in their own right.

Right ventricular myocardial infarction

Right ventricular infarction is relatively common, occurring in approximately 50% of all inferior myocardial infarcts. This is usually due to proximal thrombotic occlusion of a dominant right coronary artery. Isolated right ventricular infarction without left ventricular involvement is also recognised, but much rarer. Right ventricular infarction can cause cardiogenic shock.

Acute echo features include right ventricular dilatation, systolic impairment, regional wall motion abnormality, paradoxical septal motion and acute tricuspid regurgitation (Fig. 10.1). In the long term, echocardiographic evidence of scarring and remodelling may become apparent.

Arrhythmogenic right ventricular dysplasia (ARVD)

This is a cardiomyopathy that predominantly affects the right ventricle, though left ventricular involvement is increasingly recognised. The aetiology is unknown, but it can be familial. The right ventricular muscle is progressively replaced with fibrofatty material, leading to dilatation, and impaired function. As the name suggests, it also predisposes to ventricular arrhythmias, such as ventricular tachycardia and ventricular fibrillation.

Figure 10.1

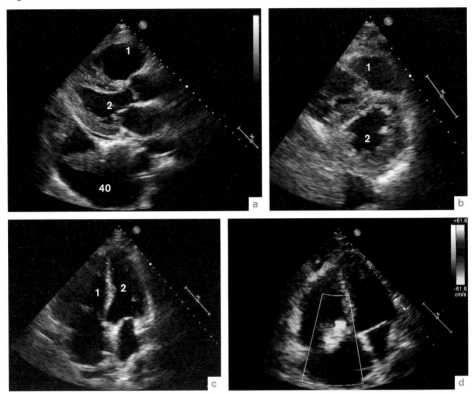

Acute right ventricular myocardial infarction. (a) Parasternal long axis view. **(b)** Parasternal short axis. **(c** and **d)** Apical four-chamber. The right ventricular free wall and inferior left ventricular wall are akinetic. The right ventricle is severely impaired, whilst overall left ventricular function is well preserved. Acute dilatation and volume overload have led to severe low-pressure tricuspid regurgitation. A pleural effusion is present.

View **On-line** Images

   Echocardiographically, the appearance ranges from evidence of mild right ventricular dilatation, to severely abnormal architecture, with deep clefts and microaneurysms in the right ventricular wall and gross dilatation/impairment (Fig. 10.2). However it is not possible to exclude the diagnosis of arrhythmogenic right ventricular cardiomyopathy on echo as subtle abnormalities may not be detectable in the early stages: magnetic resonance imaging is more sensitive and specific in this setting.

Cor pulmonale

Cor pulmonale describes the remodelling of the right ventricle in response to pulmonary hypertension, in the absence of left heart dysfunction. A wide range of

Figure 10.2

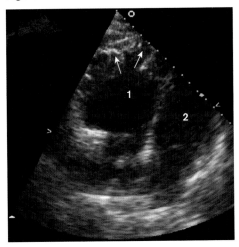

Arrhythmogenic right ventricular cardiomyopathy. Apical four-chamber view. The right ventricle is dilated and deep crevasses are present in the free wall (arrows).

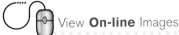 View **On-line** Images

Table 10.1 Causes of pulmonary hypertension

Group I: Pulmonary artery hypertension

Primary pulmonary hypertension: idiopathic or familial

Secondary (e.g. connective tissue disease, congenital heart disease, portal hypertension, HIV infection, drugs)

Group II: Pulmonary venous hypertension

Secondary to left-sided valvular/atrial/ventricular disease

Group III: Pulmonary hypertension secondary to respiratory disorders or hypoxia

(e.g. COPD, interstitial lung disease, obstructive sleep apnoea)

Group IV: Pulmonary hypertension secondary to thromboembolic disease

Based on the World Health Organization classification of pulmonary hypertension.
HIV, human immunodeficiency virus; COPD, chronic obstructive pulmonary disease.

pathologies can cause this (Table 10.1), but there are no specific distinguishing echocardiographic features.

Acute cor pulmonale: acute pulmonary embolism

The commonest cause of acute cor pulmonale is acute massive pulmonary embolism: this occurs when a large thrombus obstructs a major pulmonary artery, causing a sudden and severe rise in pulmonary artery pressure and pulmonary vascular resistance. In the face of this, the right ventricle effectively fails to function, becoming dilated and hypokinetic. Acute cor pulmonale can also be seen in

Figure 10.3

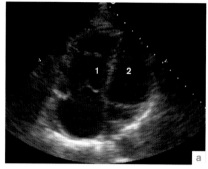
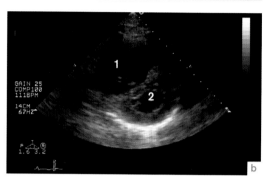
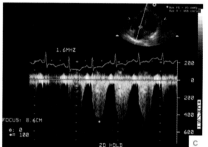
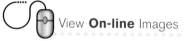

Acute pulmonary embolism. (a) Apical four-chamber view. **(b)** Parasternal short axis. **(c)** Tricuspid continuous wave Doppler. There is severe dilatation of the right ventricle, and paradoxical movement of the septum due to pressure overload. Apical right ventricular function is preserved, but otherwise function is severely impaired. Paradoxical septal motion is apparent due to severe pressure overload (right ventricular systolic pressure = 95 mmHg).

View **On-line** Images

other acute respiratory illnesses, such as acute respiratory distress syndrome, where severe hypoxia causes pulmonary vasoconstriction.

Figure 10.3 demonstrates the key echocardiographic features of acute cor pulmonale: severe right ventricular dilatation, severe global right ventricular hypokinesia with preserved apical function, interventricular septal flattening, acute tricuspid regurgitation and pulmonary hypertension.

Flattening of the interventricular septum is best seen in the parasternal short axis view, and gives the left ventricle a D-shape in late systole/early diastole. This is due to two processes. Firstly, expansion of the right ventricle within the pericardial sac effectively displaces the septum towards the left ventricle. Secondly, right ventricular ejection is prolonged compared to the left ventricle, so that right ventricular pressure transiently exceeds left ventricular pressure at the end of systole/ early diastole. Dyskinetic septal movement gives the appearance that the septum contracts with the right ventricle, rather than the left ventricle.

Evidence of acute right ventricular pressure overload in the setting of suspected/ confirmed pulmonary embolism, with evidence of haemodynamic compromise, may be an indication for thrombolytic therapy to be considered. Very occasionally mobile thrombus may be seen 'in transit' in the right heart or pulmonary artery (Fig. 10.4). Persistent right ventricular dilatation after pulmonary embolism is a marker of adverse prognosis.

Figure 10.4

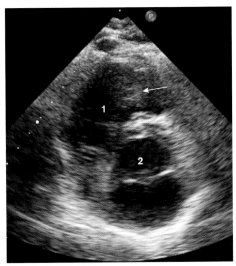

Thrombus in transit. Parasternal short axis view. A large thrombus is seen oscillating within the right ventricle of this patient with a recent history of pulmonary embolism.

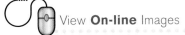

View **On-line** Images

Chronic cor pulmonale

Chronic cor pulmonale is most commonly due to chronic obstructive pulmonary disease (COPD). It is also seen with chronic thromboembolic disease and primary pulmonary hypertension. Sustained pressure overload stimulates compensatory right ventricular hypertrophy, but eventually the right ventricle dilates and fails. Volume overload may also occur due to tricuspid annular dilatation and functional tricuspid regurgitation. Again, septal flattening due to pressure/volume overload is a hallmark of this condition.

Principles of valve disease

Introduction

Heart valves are designed to permit unidirectional blood flow between cardiac chambers, with minimal resistance to forward flow. Valvular dysfunction occurs when there is obstruction to flow, regurgitation, or a mixture of both.

The assessment of valve function is a routine part of every echo examination. A great deal of information can be obtained from the general appearance of a valve, but detailed assessment requires the use of a variety of Doppler techniques. This chapter will discuss the physiological principles that apply universally to the assessment of all valves and all lesions. This provides a basis for the approach to specific valves in subsequent chapters. A similar approach can be applied to the assessment of intracardiac shunts and this will also be discussed.

Doppler techniques allow the speed, timing and direction of blood flow to be measured with great accuracy. However, it is often more useful to know about pressure gradients or volumes of blood flow across valves, neither of which can be measured directly with echo. Fortunately, a variety of methods can be used to estimate these parameters from Doppler data.

Estimating pressure gradients: the Bernoulli equation

Pressure gradients occur whenever there is a connection between heart chambers or blood vessels that are at different pressures (Fig. 11.1). Such gradients occur with any regurgitant or stenotic valve lesion, as well as intracardiac shunts, because there are almost always pressure differences between the cardiac chambers or major vessels at any one time.

Figure 11.1

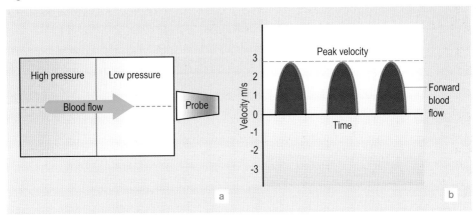

Measuring pressure gradients. (a) If two heart chambers at different pressures are connected, blood flows from the high- to low-pressure chamber (blue arrow). Aligning a Doppler beam with the blood flow allows the velocity to be measured. **(b)** The Doppler spectrum of blood flow towards the echo probe shows that the blood accelerates to a peak velocity, and then decelerates with each cardiac cycle. The peak velocity is used to calculate the pressure gradient: gradient = $4 \times 3^2 = 36$ mmHg.

Blood will flow from one chamber to another at a velocity related to the pressure difference. This is influenced by the physical properties of blood, particularly its ability to accelerate, so the exact relationship between velocity of blood flow and pressure gradients is complex. However, in most clinical situations it can be estimated from the simplified Bernoulli equation:

Pressure gradient (mmHg) = $4V^2$

where V = peak velocity (m/s).

Peak instantaneous and mean gradients

The pressure gradient is simply the pressure difference between two chambers at a specific point in time. Apart from this no other information can be inferred, and it does not tell us the actual pressure of either chamber.

Since the heart continuously cycles between contraction and relaxation, pressure gradients vary from moment to moment, depending on the precise point at which the velocity is measured. For this, and other reasons, gradients estimated by echo often differ from estimates using other methods. For example, the peak-to-peak pressure difference across a stenotic aortic valve measured directly by cardiac catheterisation is usually lower than echo estimates of the pressure gradient derived from the peak velocity. The main reason for this is that the greatest pressure difference does not occur when the peak pressure is reached, but during the pressure rise. This is known as the peak instantaneous gradient, and coincides with the peak velocity (Fig. 11.2).

Peak velocity is easy to identify and is reproducible, making it the routine method for assessing gradients across the aortic valve, left ventricular outflow tract (LVOT), pulmonary valve, interventricular shunts and tricuspid valve.

Figure 11.2

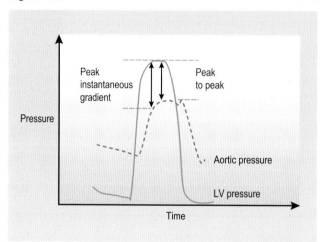

Different measurements of aortic stenosis gradient. In the presence of aortic stenosis the systolic pressures in the left ventricle (LV) (blue line) and aorta (red line) are markedly different, creating a pressure gradient. Cardiac catheterisation can measure the difference between the peak aortic pressure and the peak left ventricular pressure, though these do not occur absolutely simultaneously. In contrast echocardiographic measurement of the peak velocity of blood flow across the aortic valve estimates the maximal gradient driving blood flow across the stenosis at any one moment. This is otherwise known as the peak instantaneous gradient, and is generally greater than the peak-to-peak gradient.

Figure 11.3

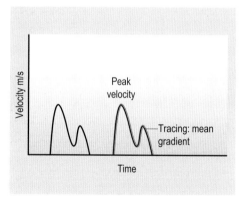

Mean pressure gradient. The mean gradient across a valve can be calculated by tracing the envelope of the Doppler spectrum as illustrated (red line). Although this method can be applied to any valve, it is particularly useful when the blood flow pattern is complex (e.g. transmitral diastolic flow).

When blood flow is complex, the mean gradient may be more relevant than the peak (Fig. 11.3). This is calculated by measuring the velocity at all time points during blood flow and dividing by the duration of flow. In practical terms this simply involves tracing the velocity envelope of the Doppler spectrum, and the mean gradient is automatically computed by the echo machine.

Mean gradients are used for assessing stenotic lesions, particularly at the aortic and mitral valves.

Measuring volumes and flow

Quantitative echocardiography is a method of estimating volumes of blood flow from velocity data. This is not as difficult as may first appear. Consider a very simple situation in which blood flows through a long tube at a constant velocity (Fig. 11.4). If we know the velocity of flow, then we can work out how far along the tube the blood will travel over a particular time period (distance travelled = velocity × time). From this we can work out the volume of blood flowing past a reference point in the tube by measuring the cross-sectional area at the same point.

Volume = distance × cross-sectional area

so

Volume = velocity × time × cross-sectional area

The situation in the heart is more complex because flow is pulsatile, so the velocity is constantly changing. To estimate the volume of blood accurately we need to take into account all the different velocities with the duration of flow at each velocity: this is known as the velocity time integral (VTI). The VTI is in fact equal to the area of the Doppler spectrum, so simply tracing the edge of the velocity envelope from the baseline back to the baseline allows the area to be calculated (Fig. 11.5).

If we know the VTI at a specific structure through which blood passes, measurement of the cross-sectional area at that point allows the volume of blood flow to be calculated. In most situations it is possible to choose circular structures (e.g. vessels and valve annulus) so that we can estimate cross-sectional area simply by measuring the diameter of the structure (area of circle = π × radius²). Therefore,

Volume of blood flow = VTI × cross-sectional area

Volume of blood flow = VTI × π × radius²

In principle, flow volumes can be calculated from VTI data and cross-sectional diameter measurements at any site in the heart or great vessels where the orifice/conduit is circular and the diameter is fixed. Suitable sites include the LVOT, right ventricular outflow tract (RVOT), mitral valve annulus and great vessels. The

Figure 11.4

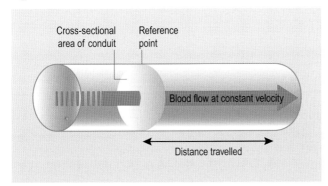

Cross-sectional area of conduit

Reference point

Blood flow at constant velocity

Distance travelled

Calculating blood flow volume from velocity data. If blood flows along a cylindrical conduit at a constant velocity (red arrow) the volume of blood passing a reference point in the cylinder over a certain time is equal to the distance travelled by the blood in that time, multiplied by the cross-sectional area of the conduit.

Figure 11.5

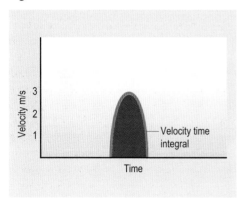

Velocity time integral. Velocity time integral is measured by tracing round the Doppler spectrum (red line) from baseline back to baseline. The area under the curve (black) equals the velocity time integral and can be used for calculations.

Table 11.1 Technical recommendations for measurements of stroke volume

Site	Parameter	Method
LVOT	SV_{LV}	LVOT diameter: maximum diameter just prior to AV annulus in mid-systole from PSLAX view
		PW Doppler: sample volume just prior to AV in A5C view
RVOT	SV_{RV}	RVOT diameter: maximum diameter just prior to PV annulus in PSSAX view in mid-systole
		PW Doppler: sample volume just prior to PV annulus in PSSAX view
MV annulus		Mitral annular diameter: maximum diameter in early diastole in A4C view
		Or mitral annular area: PSSAX view: trace annular area in early diastole
		PW Doppler: sample volume in line with MV annulus in A4C view (i.e. not at MV tips)

The tricuspid valve is rarely used in practice and is not included.
LVOT, left ventricular outflow tract; SV, stroke volume; AV, aortic valve; PSLAX, parasternal long axis; PW, pulse wave; A5C, apical five-chamber; RVOT, right ventricular outflow tract; PV, pulmonary valve; PSSAX, parasternal short axis; A4C, apical four-chamber; MV, mitral valve.

aortic and pulmonary valve orifices cannot be used because they are not circular, whilst measurements at the tricuspid annulus can be unreliable.

Blood flows through the LVOT and RVOT are actually the same as the stroke volumes of the left and right ventricles, respectively (i.e. volume of blood ejected during each cardiac cycle). Therefore cardiac output is obtained by multiplying the stroke volume by the heart rate.

The methods for assessing blood flow at the LVOT, RVOT and mitral valve annulus are summarised in Table 11.1.

Clinical applications: continuity and discontinuity

Quantitative echo techniques can be applied to a variety of situations, including estimation of aortic valve area, shunt ratios, and valvular regurgitant volume or fraction.

These applications are based on the principle that the heart is a closed system, so that the volume of blood entering the right heart and leaving the left heart should be constant. Therefore, flow volumes across all valves and through all chambers should be exactly equal. In other words, there is conservation of matter. Conversely, if there is a significant difference in the outputs of the left and right sides of the heart ('discontinuity'), there must be an intracardiac shunt or significant valvular leak. Consequently, if we can measure the blood flow across one valve we can use this information to interpret changes in blood flow across another valve or shunt.

Estimation of valve area: the continuity equation

The continuity equation is routinely used to estimate aortic valve area in aortic stenosis. It is based on the assumption that the volume of blood pumped through the LVOT during each cardiac cycle (left ventricular stroke volume) is the same as the volume of blood crossing the aortic valve. We have already seen that the transaortic blood flow volume is equal to the product of the LVOT VTI and LVOT area.

Volume leaving outflow tract = volume ejected through aortic valve (AV)

$$\text{Area}_{LVOT} \times \text{VTI}_{LVOT} = \text{area}_{AV} \times \text{VTI}_{AV}$$

$$\text{Area}_{AV} = (\text{area}_{LVOT} \times \text{VTI}_{LVOT})/\text{VTI}_{AV}$$

$$\text{Area}_{AV} = [(\pi\ \text{radius}_{LVOT}{}^2) \times \text{VTI}_{LVOT}]\text{VTI}_{AV}$$

The measurements required for this method are illustrated schematically in Figure 11.6, and its clinical application is discussed in more detail in Chapter 12. It is worth noting that a simplified approach using peak velocity measurements in the LVOT and aortic valve rather than VTI measurements can be used instead.

Regurgitant fraction: discontinuity

If we know that a valve is regurgitant, the forward flow across all valves will no longer be equal. We can use this discrepancy to determine the severity of regurgitation by estimating the differences in flow volumes at two different sites in the heart. The proportional difference between forward flows at two valves is the regurgitant fraction.

This is best understood by considering an example, such as a case of severe mitral regurgitation. During systole the left ventricle ejects blood through the LVOT and aortic valve into the systemic circulation. In the presence of severe mitral regurgitation a significant volume of blood is also ejected back into the left

Figure 11.6

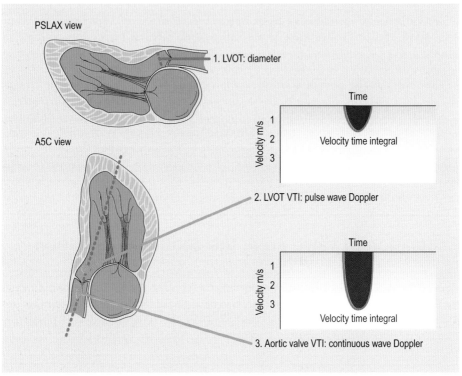

Measurements required for the continuity equation. 1, Left ventricular outflow tract (LVOT) diameter is measured from the parasternal long axis (PSLAX) view (green line). 2, Pulse wave Doppler is used for LVOT velocity time integral (VTI). 3, Continuous wave Doppler is used for aortic valve VTI. A5C, apical five-chamber.

atrium. The difference between the volume of blood filling the ventricle in diastole and the volume ejected through the LVOT in systole (stroke volume) is the mitral regurgitant volume.

Left ventricular stroke volume can be measured as described above, whilst left ventricular diastolic volume can be estimated by measuring blood flow from the left atrium through the mitral valve annulus in diastole. Regurgitant fraction is the regurgitant volume expressed as a percentage of the total forward flow across that valve.

Regurgitant volume = transmitral inflow volume − left ventricular stroke volume

Regurgitant fraction = (regurgitant volume/transmitral inflow volume) × 100

Theoretically the same techniques can be applied to regurgitation of any valve, as long as it is possible to obtain reliable estimates of flow at two different sites in the heart, and there are no shunts. In practice the right and left ventricular stroke volumes are the favoured sites of measurement because these can be measured more reliably than flow at the mitral or tricuspid valves.

Potential limitations

The greatest limitation of quantitative echo techniques is operator error. Significant inaccuracies can be introduced by errors in measuring the conduit diameter, poor Doppler alignment and failure to make these measurements at the exact same location. Most of all, experience and practice are required to become competent at these techniques. It is a good idea to practise on normal subjects to check the accuracy of your technique: flow volumes at different sites should be equal. It is also sensible to check the compatibility of quantitative data with other echo parameters.

The presence of multiple pathologies can invalidate or at least complicate calculations. For reliable estimates of valvular regurgitation there should not be an intracardiac shunt, or vice versa. Finally, atrial fibrillation can cause significant beat-to-beat variability, so multiple beats (>5) should be analysed, and the average taken.

Effective regurgitant orifice area: PISA

The principles of the continuity equation can be applied to quantitative analysis of regurgitant valve lesions to estimate the size of the valve defect causing regurgitation. This is known as the effective regurgitant orifice area (EROA), and can be used as a measure of regurgitation severity.

Blood flow across a regurgitant valve orifice is very similar to blood flow across a stenotic valve. In both cases there is initial acceleration and convergence of flow around the valve orifice, reaching a peak velocity as blood transits the valve. Immediately after passing through the valve orifice the jet is at its narrowest, and this is known as the vena contracta. The jet then widens as adjacent blood is recruited to flow with the jet.

Flow convergence can be seen on colour flow mapping (CFM) Doppler as a semicircular coloured area around a valve orifice (Fig. 11.7). When the velocity of blood accelerating towards the valve exceeds the velocity range measurable by CFM Doppler (Nyquist limit, or aliasing velocity), there is an abrupt change in the computer-assigned colouring of blood flow. This creates the appearance of a distinct semicircular zone, with the valve orifice at the centre. The point at which colour change/aliasing occurs depends on the velocity settings used, and this will determine the apparent size of the flow convergence zone. Of course the echo depicts a two-dimensional representation of blood flow, but in reality the convergence zone is a hemisphere with an outer rim defined by the aliasing velocity. All points on this hemisphere have the same velocity, so it is known as the proximal isovelocity surface area (PISA). The abrupt colour change at the PISA makes it clearly identifiable, but it is just one of multiple concentric isovelocity 'shells' that converge on the valve orifice. If you imagine an onion cut in half, each layer represents an isovelocity shell, and the transition between the onion skin and flesh represents the PISA.

The continuity equation can be applied to work out the EROA because we can treat the flow convergence zone as though it is an orifice or conduit funnelling blood towards the valve orifice, analogous to the LVOT. The continuity equation in this situation is as follows:

Figure 11.7

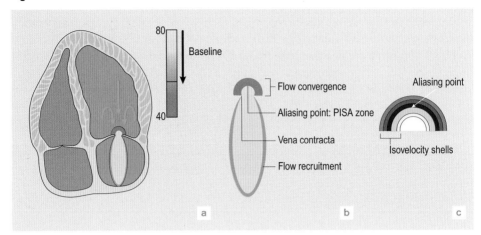

Regurgitant blood flow. (a and b) Colour flow mapping (CFM) Doppler of mitral regurgitation is represented schematically in an apical four-chamber view. During systole, blood is forced towards the mitral valve (blue arrows) and converges on the regurgitant orifice (blue halo). As blood accelerates towards the orifice the Doppler signal abruptly changes to yellow at the aliasing point. This represents the hemispheric proximal isovelocity surface area (PISA). As blood travels through the orifice, flow becomes turbulent and it reaches its maximal velocity. The narrow portion of the jet just after the orifice is the vena contracta. The regurgitant jet also recruits blood in the left atrium to flow backwards (flow recruitment: orange). Note that the CFM Doppler settings have been adjusted to maximise the size of the PISA zone and the colour contrast at this point by reducing the aliasing velocity to 40 cm/s, and shifting the colour scale baseline to make it two-tone. **(c)** The flow convergence zone comprises multiple concentric isovelocity shells that centre on the valve orifice.

$$\text{PISA} \times \text{aliasing velocity } (V_a) = \text{EROA} \times \text{peak velocity } (V_{max})$$

$$\text{The surface area of the proximal isovelocity shell} = 2\pi r^2$$

where r is the radius of the PISA shell, measured from the aliasing point to the centre of the regurgitant orifice. Therefore,

$$(2\pi r^2) \times V_a = \text{EROA} \times V_{max}$$

$$\text{EROA} = [(2\pi r^2) \times V_a]/V_{max}$$

So to calculate EROA we need to measure three things:
1. the radius of the PISA hemisphere
2. the aliasing velocity of the PISA
3. the maximum velocity of blood flow through the valve orifice.

Although the continuity equation described previously relied on VTI measurements, this is not possible with CFM Doppler, and peak velocities provide a satisfactory substitute.

Finally, to estimate the regurgitant volume, we must calculate the flow through the regurgitant valve by measuring the VTI of the flow through the valve from the continuous wave Doppler trace.

Hence, regurgitant volume = EROA × VTI$_{max}$.

PISA in practice: an example

To obtain good-quality images of flow convergence for PISA analysis, the following steps are recommended (Figs 11.7 and 11.8):

1. Use a view that shows the convergence zone optimally, e.g. apical four-chamber for mitral regurgitant jets (Fig. 11.8a).
2. Magnify the area of interest (Fig. 11.8b)
3. Maximise the size of the PISA shell by adjusting the Doppler scale so that the aliasing velocity (V_a) is set around 40 cm/s. This is best done by adjusting the baseline of the Doppler scale, so that the colour spectrum becomes two-tone, thereby enhancing the colour contrast at the PISA. This makes the CFM scale asymmetric with different aliasing velocities at either end of the scale. The scale should be altered in the direction of the regurgitant jet. Obtaining an exact value of 40 cm/s may require adjustment of the image depth.

Figure 11.8

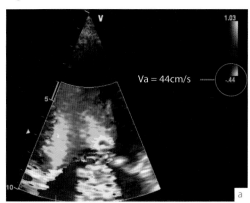

Va = 44cm/s   .44

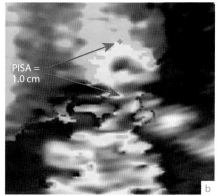

PISA = 1.0 cm

a

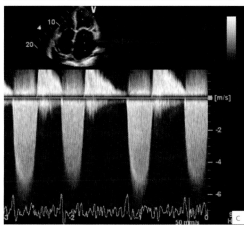

[m/s]

-2

-4

-6

50 mm/s

c

Mitral regurgitation: proximal isovelocity surface area (PISA) calculation. (a) Colour flow mapping (CFM) Doppler demonstrating a central jet of mitral regurgitation. The baseline of the CFM velocity scale has been adjusted so that the lower aliasing velocity is 44 cm/s. **(b)** CFM Doppler (magnified). The PISA radius is measured from the aliasing point (junction of the blue/yellow interface) to the centre of the mitral valve orifice (use the 'colour suppress' option to reveal the orifice of the mitral valve). **(c)** Continuous wave Doppler through the vena contracta of the mitral regurgitation jet. $V_{max} = 600$ cm/s.
Effective regurgitant orifice area =
$2\pi r^2 \times V_a/V_{max} = 6.284 \times 1.0^2 \times 44/600 = 0.46$ cm^2. This indicates severe mitral regurgitation (>0.4 cm^2).

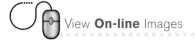

View **On-line** Images

4. Measure the radius of the PISA zone. To do this, freeze the image on the frame that shows the maximal PISA size in mid-systole, and place a cursor on the aliasing point, perpendicular to the valve orifice. Next, use the 'colour suppress' option to reveal the two-dimensional image of the valve, which is otherwise obscured by the colour flow image. This enables you to identify the valve orifice accurately.

5. Make continuous wave Doppler measurements through the valve orifice, to obtain the peak velocity (V_{max}).

Potential limitations

Because many assumptions are used to calculate PISA, there is potential for misleading estimates of EROA and regurgitant volume. For example, the regurgitant orifice may not be circular at all, or there may be more than one regurgitant jet. In addition, it can be difficult to decide exactly where to make measurements if the picture quality is suboptimal, or if the PISA is not well defined or is a non-uniform shape. The PISA size actually varies as systole progresses, and the maximal radius should be chosen as this coincides with the timing of the peak velocity measurement that is used. Eccentric jets can also be problematic, because the zone of flow convergence may be non-hemispheric, and it can be difficult to obtain an accurate V_{max}. Nevertheless, this technique is increasingly used to assess valve regurgitation.

The aortic valve

The normal aortic valve

The aortic valve has three semilunar cusps that allow unidirectional blood flow out of the left ventricle into the aorta. The cusps are thin and fibrous, and attach at their bases to the aortic ring. The cusps are named according to the coronary artery that originates from adjacent sinus of Valsalva: left, right and non-coronary.

Echocardiographic appearance

The cusps of a healthy aortic valve are thin (<2 mm), slightly echo-bright and mobile. In the parasternal long axis (PSLAX) view a single central closure line is seen (Fig. 12.1). The leaflets should pivot through approximately 90°, so that the minimum tip separation is at least 2 cm in mid-systole. In the parasternal short axis (PSSAX) view the valve is seen *en face*, and three cusps are visible, forming a 'Mercedes Benz' pattern in diastole (Fig. 12.1c). This appearance is also seen in the subcostal short axis view.

Doppler examination

Blood flow across the aortic valve should be routinely assessed from the apical five-chamber (A5C) view using colour flow mapping (CFM) and continuous wave (CW) Doppler aligned with blood flow. Flow is laminar, with rapid acceleration, reaching a peak velocity of around 1 m/s (normal <1.7 m/s) (Fig. 12.2). Aortic regurgitation should not be detectable.

Aortic valve sclerosis

Aortic valve sclerosis is a degenerative condition in which there is thickening and calcification of the aortic valve leaflets

Figure 12.1

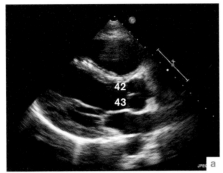

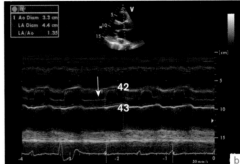

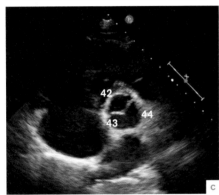

Normal aortic valve. (a) Parasternal long axis (PSLAX). (b) M-mode. (c) Parasternal short axis (PSSAX). The right and non-coronary cusps of the aortic valve are seen in the PSLAX view and M-mode. The closure line is central within the aortic root (arrow). In the PSSAX view the three cusps are clearly seen.

View **On-line** Images

Figure 12.2

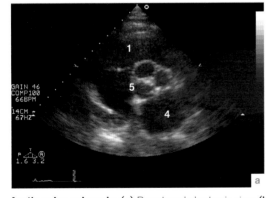

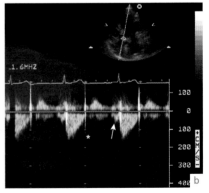

Aortic valve sclerosis. (a) Parasternal short axis view. (b) Transaortic continuous wave Doppler. The aortic valve cusps are thickened and echogenic at the tips. However, there is no significant haemodynamic gradient across the aortic valve. The continuous wave Doppler spectrum demonstrates pre-ejection velocities caused by atrial contraction/isovolumic left ventricular contraction (arrow) as well as aortic valve closure signals (*). These are normal.

(Fig. 12.2). It may occur as a localised or diffuse process. In contrast to aortic stenosis there is no obstruction to blood flow (peak velocity <1.7 m/s), cusp mobility is preserved and the condition is benign. It is an important cause of aortic murmurs in the elderly and is therefore a common cause for echo referral.

Aortic valve stenosis

Aortic stenosis is characterised by obstruction of blood flow through the aortic valve, due to reduced cusp excursion. The valve is usually highly calcified, thickened and immobile. Calcific degeneration of a normal trileaflet aortic valve can be thought of as part of a normal ageing process: patients typically present after 60 years of age. Bicuspid aortic valves are subject to abnormal mechanical stresses and blood flow, leading to accelerated calcific degeneration: patients typically present between 30 and 50 years of age. Rheumatic aortic valve disease is rare in Western societies, but is the commonest cause of aortic stenosis worldwide: rheumatic valve disease is considered in more detail in Chapter 13.

Aortic valve area is normally 3–4 cm² in adults, depending on body size. A significant obstruction does not occur until there is a reduction in valve area of approximately 70%. The haemodynamic effects of aortic stenosis can lead to angina, heart failure, left ventricular hypertrophy (LVH) and syncope. It is, therefore, an important diagnosis to make because aortic valve replacement significantly improves the prognosis of patients with symptomatic severe aortic stenosis.

Echocardiographic appearance

The appearance of aortic stenosis on two-dimensional imaging depends on the severity of stenosis, and the underlying aetiology. With severe aortic stenosis the cusps are usually highly calcified, appearing thickened and much brighter than other structures. Mobility is reduced, or almost non-existent, resulting in a small or barely discernible orifice during systole (Fig. 12.4). Not surprisingly the appearance of valves with a lesser degree of stenosis is less abnormal (Fig. 12.3).

Calcific degeneration tends to result in nodules of calcium forming around the annulus and spreading into the base/body of the cusps, leaving the free edges unaffected. By contrast rheumatic degeneration causes commissural fusion and thickening/retraction of the tips: it is almost always associated with rheumatic mitral valve disease. However, with advanced disease it may be impossible to discern the underlying aetiology. The appearance of bicuspid valves is discussed in a later section.

Assessment of aortic stenosis

There are three ways of assessing the severity of aortic stenosis:
1. Aortic valve gradient
2. Estimation of aortic valve area
3. Planimetry of aortic valve orifice

Figure 12.3

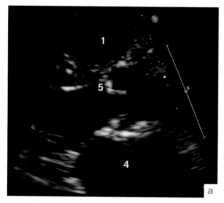

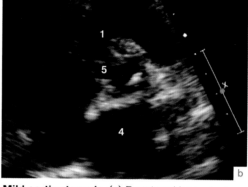

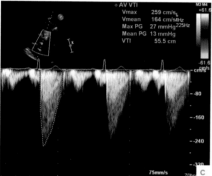

AV VTI		M3 M4
Vmax	259 cm/s	+61.6
Vmean	164 cm/s	225Hz
Max PG	27 mmHg	
Mean PG	13 mmHg	
VTI	55.5 cm	

Mild aortic stenosis. (a) Parasternal long axis view (mid-systole). **(b)** Parasternal short axis view (mid-systole). **(c)** Transaortic valve continuous wave Doppler. The aortic valve cusps are mildly calcified, resulting in gradient of 27 mmHg. Cusp mobility is particularly restricted at the bases.

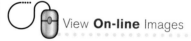 View **On-line** Images

Aortic valve gradient

Simplified Bernoulli equation

The principles of the simplified Bernoulli equation were discussed in Chapter 11. Essentially, aortic valve obstruction creates a pressure gradient between the left ventricle and aorta, leading to acceleration of blood flow as it crosses the aortic valve. The increase in blood velocity is measured to estimate the valve gradient using the formula:

Peak instantaneous pressure gradient $= 4 \times$ peak velocity^2

This method is routinely applied to the assessment of aortic stenosis. It requires measurement of the transaortic peak velocity from a good-quality A5C view using CW Doppler aligned with transaortic blood flow. In this view, aortic outflow is away from the probe, and is therefore represented below the baseline on the Doppler trace (Fig. 12.3). The cursor is used to measure the peak velocity, and most echo machines will automatically calculate the peak instantaneous gradient. Mean gradient can also be measured by tracing around the velocity envelope, as described in Chapter 11.

Figure 12.4

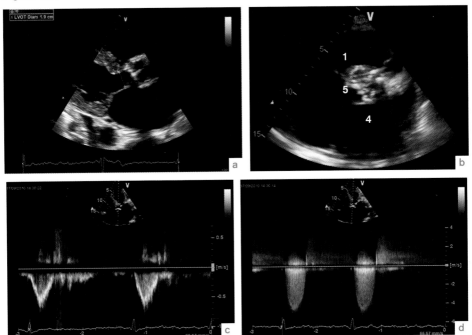

Severe aortic stenosis secondary to degenerative calcification. (a) Parasternal long axis view. (b) Parasternal short axis view. (c) Left ventricular outflow tract (LVOT) pulse wave Doppler. (d) Transaortic continuous wave Doppler. $V_{LVOT} = 76$ cm/s; $V_{AV} = 534$ cm/s; $VTI_{LVOT} = 18$ cm; $VTI_{AV} = 139$ cm; LVOT diameter = 1.9 cm. VTI, velocity time integral. Calcific degeneration renders the aortic valve almost immobile. Doppler assessment confirms severe aortic stenosis. Aortic valve gradient = 114 mmHg. Mean gradient = 74 mmHg. Aortic valve area = 0.4 cm^2 (using both the peak velocity and VTI methods). Ratio of velocities = 0.14.

View **On-line** Images

Pitfalls

Underestimation of the peak velocity is common if the Doppler cursor is not properly aligned with blood flow: this may be suspected if the signal appears weak, or the spectral envelope is incomplete. If a patient is in atrial fibrillation the peak velocity can be quite variable, so the average of 3–5 beats should be taken.

Although the multipurpose echo probe generally provides adequate information, some echocardiography machines are equipped with a dedicated stand-alone Doppler probe (Pedoff probe) that gives more accurate CW Doppler data (Fig. 12.5). This is used from both the apical view and a right parasternal view (second intercostal space, with the patient lying vertically on the right-hand side).

It is important to appreciate that Doppler measurements only provide an estimate of the pressure gradient and may be wrong. In fact, the simplified Bernoulli equation only applies if left ventricular systolic function is normal, and the velocity of blood in the left ventricular outflow tract (LVOT) is approximately 1 m/s. Peak velocity may be spuriously increased if left ventricular function is hyperdynamic

Figure 12.5

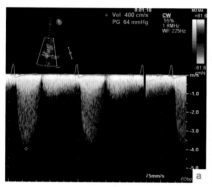
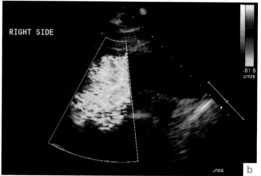

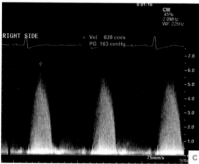
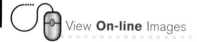

Assessing aortic valve gradient from the right parasternal view. **(a)** A peak gradient of 64 mmHg was recorded with the multipurpose probe from the apical position. **(b)** Right parasternal view of ascending aorta showing jet of high-velocity blood flow. **(c)** A peak gradient of 163 mmHg was recorded in the same patient from a right parasternal position using a stand-alone Doppler probe.

View **On-line** Images

(e.g. severe aortic regurgitation, post ventricular ectopic beat) or decreased (e.g. severe left ventricular dysfunction). It is also important to avoid eccentric jets of mitral or tricuspid regurgitation, which can be confused with the aortic valve signal. Finally it is worth remembering that CW Doppler does not localise the site of obstruction and it is possible that coexisting sub- or supravalvular obstruction may also contribute to a gradient.

Estimation of aortic valve area

The continuity equation
The theoretical basis of the continuity equation has been discussed in Chapter 11. It should be used routinely to assess aortic valve area, particularly if left ventricular stroke volume is abnormally low or high, as this is taken into account by measuring blood flow in the LVOT.

Calculation of aortic valve area requires measurement of the velocity time integral (VTI) of blood flow in the LVOT and across the aortic valve with pulse wave (PW) and CW Doppler, respectively. LVOT diameter is measured from the PSLAX view on two-dimensional images. Be sure to use the LVOT radius and not the diameter! The methodology is illustrated in Figures 11.6 and 12.4. Most echo software packages will calculate the aortic valve area automatically from the relevant parameters.

$$Area_{AV} = (area_{LVOT} \times VTI_{LVOT})/VTI_{AV}$$

$$Area_{AV} = [(\pi\, radius_{LVOT}{}^2) \times VTI_{LVOT}]/VTI_{AV}$$

Since blood is not ejected at a constant velocity it is theoretically better to use the VTI, but in practice using the peak velocity actually works just as well.

Pitfalls

Aortic valve area is an estimate, and relies very heavily on measuring the LVOT diameter accurately. Small errors of measurement are magnified by the calculation of area data from a single linear measurement. If LVOT is difficult to measure with confidence it is preferable simply to quote the ratio of the aortic valve and LVOT peak velocities (Table 12.1 and Fig. 12.4). This will allow LVOT blood flow to be taken into account without the risk of introducing significant errors. A ratio <0.25 suggests severe aortic stenosis.

In very low cardiac output states the continuity equation may underestimate the valve area so that there appears to be severe aortic stenosis (valve area <1 cm²) with a low gradient (<30 mmHg). In this situation it can be difficult to tell if there is true severe aortic stenosis (low-gradient aortic stenosis) causing heart failure, which may be amenable to aortic valve replacement, or if there is an unrelated cardiomyopathy with mild-to-moderate aortic stenosis. Dobutamine stress echo may be helpful by assessing the effect of increased cardiac output on valve parameters. An increase in peak velocity (>0.6 m/s) or peak gradient (>20 mmHg increase) with minimal change in aortic valve area (<20% increase) suggests that aortic stenosis is severe. Conversely, a smaller rise in velocity/gradient with a rise in valve area (>25%) suggests that stenosis is not severe.

Aortic valve planimetry

Direct measurement of aortic valve area can be performed if high-quality cross-sectional images of the aortic valve can be obtained at the tips of the valve cusps.

Table 12.1 Severity of aortic stenosis

Parameter	Mild	Moderate	Severe
Valve area (cm²)	>1.5	1.5–1.0	<1.0*
Peak velocity (m/s)	2.6–2.9	3.0–4.0	>4.0
Ratio of velocities	>0.5	0.25–0.50	<0.25
Peak gradient (mmHg)	16–36	37–64	>64
Mean gradient (mmHg)	<20	20–40	>40

*Some authorities use a lower limit of 0.75 cm².

Figure 12.6

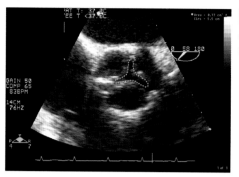

Planimetry of the aortic valve area.
Transoesophageal echo at the level of the aortic valve. Planimetered area is 0.77 cm², suggesting severe aortic stenosis.

Failure to align correctly with the tips will lead to an overestimate of valve area. In practice this requires transoesophageal echo/three-dimensional echo (Fig. 12.6). The area of the aortic valve orifice is traced in systole. Heavy calcification can obscure the orifice, leading to inaccuracy.

Assessment of the left ventricle

The left ventricle should be assessed along standard lines to define left ventricular dimensions, mass, systolic and diastolic function. Aortic stenosis causes pressure overload of the left ventricle, invariably leading to LVH and diastolic dysfunction. Therefore the absence of LVH should cast doubt on a diagnosis of severe aortic stenosis. Systolic dysfunction and left ventricular dilatation usually occur late in the natural history of aortic stenosis, so significant left ventricular dysfunction disproportionate to the severity of valvular disease suggests the presence of a coexisting cardiomyopathy. In general, LVH and left ventricular dysfunction can improve after aortic valve replacement, but severe left ventricular remodelling may not resolve completely.

Surgery for aortic stenosis

Aortic valve replacement is considered in patients with echocardiographic criteria of severe aortic stenosis and symptoms of limiting breathlessness, angina or unexplained syncope. Asymptomatic patients are not routinely considered for surgery until symptoms develop, unless there is echocardiographic evidence of progressive left ventricular systolic dysfunction or severe LVH. Patients with lesser degrees of aortic stenosis who are undergoing heart surgery for other reasons (e.g. coronary artery bypass grafting) may be considered for simultaneous aortic valve replacement as this can avoid the need for reoperation in the future.

Aortic valve regurgitation

Aortic regurgitation is retrograde flow of blood through the aortic valve during diastole. It is always abnormal and indicates a structural problem with the aortic valve or aortic root.

Detection of aortic regurgitation

Aortic regurgitation can usually be visualised very easily with CFM Doppler in the A5C, apical three-chamber, PSLAX and PSSAX views. A quick impression can be gained about the number of jets, jet origin, orientation and severity of aortic regurgitation. It is therefore the initial method of choice for detecting and evaluating aortic regurgitation. When aortic regurgitation is detected you should ask two questions: how severe is the regurgitation, and what is the underlying cause?

Assessment of chronic aortic regurgitation severity

The severity of aortic regurgitation is determined by the size of the orifice, and the volume of regurgitant blood. This cannot be measured directly using echo, so assessment is based on surrogate measures using Doppler techniques. Certain parameters are better than others, but in reality no single measurement can be relied on completely, and many different ones have to be taken into account. Figure 12.7 summarises a suggested hierarchical approach to assessing aortic regurgitation, whilst Table 12.2 gives generally accepted values for each parameter.

Specific measures

Vena contracta

The vena contracta is the narrowest portion of the regurgitant jet after it has passed through the orifice of the valve (Fig. 12.8). It is relatively independent of the settings of the echo machine or haemodynamic variables, and as such is considered to be a robust measure of aortic regurgitation severity. It should be measured in a standardised way from a magnified PSLAX view of the aortic valve with the Nyquist limit set to 50–60 cm/s. Severe aortic regurgitation has a vena contracta diameter >0.6 cm, whereas mild is <0.3 cm. Because these values are fairly similar, small errors of measurement can easily lead to misclassification.

Figure 12.7

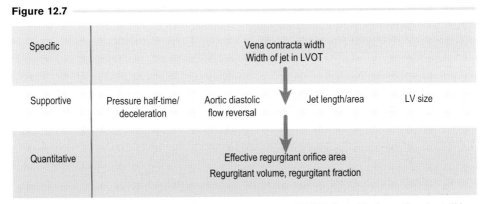

Hierarchical approach to assessing aortic regurgitation. LVOT, left ventricular outflow tract; LV, left ventricle.

Table 12.2 Severity of chronic aortic regurgitation

Parameter	Mild	Moderate	Severe
Vena contracta (cm)*	<0.3		>0.6
Jet width in LVOT*	<25%		>65%
Pressure half-time (ms)	>500		<200
Deceleration (m/s^2)	<2		>3
Aortic flow reversal	Minimal		Pan-diastolic
LV dimensions	Normal		Enlarged
EROA (cm^2)	<0.1		≥0.3
RF (%)	<30		≥50
RV (ml/beat)	<30		≥60

LVOT, left ventricular outflow tract; LV, left ventricle; EROA, effective regurgitant orifice area; RF, regurgitant fraction; RV, regurgitant volume.
*Aliasing velocity set at 50–60 cm/s.

Figure 12.8

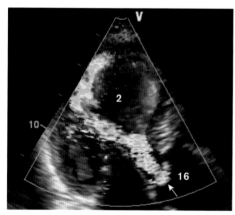

Assessment of aortic regurgitation: colour flow mapping. Three components of the jet can be identified. (1) Flow convergence zone: this is seen in red/yellow (arrow). (2) Vena contracta: the narrowest point as the jet passes through the valve orifice (between arrowheads). (3) Tail: this expands to fill most of the left ventricular outflow tract, and extends deep into the left ventricular cavity.

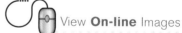 View **On-line** Images

Jet width in the LVOT

Regurgitant jet width in the LVOT is also considered a reliable measure of regurgitation severity. This is best performed in the PSLAX view using CFM and M-mode to measure both the LVOT and jet width accurately (Fig. 12.9). The widest part of the jet should be measured. A jet width greater than 60% of the LVOT diameter suggests severe regurgitation: less than 25% is evidence of mild atrial regurgitation. Difficulties can arise with very eccentric jets.

Figure 12.9

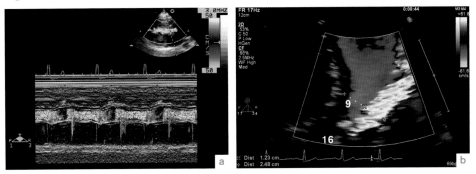

Width of jet in the left ventricular outflow tract (LVOT). (a) Assessment by colour flow M-mode across the LVOT (parasternal long axis view). **(b)** Direct measurement (apical five-chamber view).

Figure 12.10

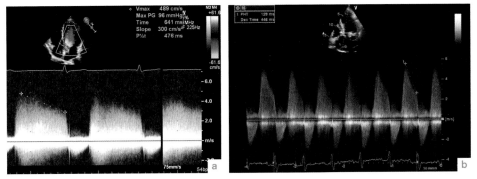

Spectral Doppler assessment of aortic regurgitation. Continuous wave Doppler from apical five-chamber view. **(a)** Mild–moderate aortic regurgitation. Pressure half-time 476 ms. **(b)** Severe aortic regurgitation. Pressure half-time 129 ms.

Supportive measures

Jet area/length

Traditionally, jet length and area have been used to assess severity. A jet that extends as far back as the left ventricular apex may be significant. Unfortunately such analysis is subject to confounding by gain/aliasing settings, Coanda effect and mixing with normal mitral inflow. This method should therefore not be relied upon.

Pressure half-time and rate of deceleration

Spectral Doppler assesses the velocity changes associated with regurgitant jets to infer information about the severity of regurgitation. A large regurgitant volume causes rapid equalisation of ventricular and aortic pressures, so that regurgitant blood flow declines rapidly. The rapid fall in velocity can be quantified by measuring either the pressure half-time or the rate of deceleration using CW Doppler (Fig. 12.10). The Doppler cursor should be aligned with the vena contracta of the regurgitant jet on CFM. Pressure half-time ($T_{1/2}$) is the time taken for the *pressure* to fall to half the peak value: since velocity is measured rather than pressure, this value is not immediately obvious from Doppler spectra. Values are given in Table 12.2.

In addition, the volume of regurgitant blood can be assessed semiquantitatively from the intensity of the regurgitant Doppler signal compared to the forward flow.

Descending aortic diastolic flow reversal

If a large volume of blood empties from the aorta back into the left ventricle, blood flow reversal will also be detectable further down the aorta. This can be examined using the suprasternal view, with PW Doppler interrogation in the descending aorta (Fig. 12.11). Significant flow reversal lasts throughout diastole.

Quantitative echocardiographic techniques

Quantitative techniques can be used to estimate the volume of regurgitant blood, or the regurgitant fraction. Aortic regurgitation increases the diastolic volume of the left ventricle, leading to an increased stroke volume compared to that of the right ventricle. The difference between these is the regurgitant volume, and this can be expressed as a fraction of the left ventricular stroke volume (regurgitant fraction). Left and right ventricular stroke volumes are measured as described in Chapter 11. In practice this type of analysis requires experience and is not routinely performed.

Regurgitant volume = left ventricular stroke volume − right ventricular stroke volume

Regurgitant fraction = regurgitant volume/left ventricular stroke volume

Figure 12.11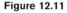

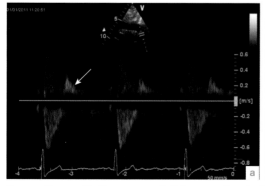 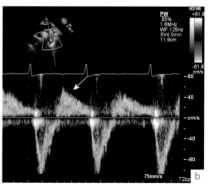

Descending aortic flow reversal. Pulse wave Doppler in the descending aorta. Aortic regurgitation causes diastolic flow reversal (arrows). **(a)** Mild−moderate aortic regurgitation: minimal diastolic flow reversal. **(b)** Severe aortic regurgitation: pan-diastolic flow reversal.

Effective regurgitant orifice area (EROA)

The concepts of proximal isovelocity surface area (PISA) have been discussed previously in Chapter 11. Appreciable flow convergence suggests that severe aortic regurgitation may be present (Fig. 12.8). Effective regurgitant orifice area can be estimated from the size of the PISA radius in early diastole, the aliasing velocity and peak regurgitant velocity (see Chapter 11). EROA ≥ 0.3 cm^2 is considered severe.

Assessment of the left ventricle in chronic aortic regurgitation

Chronic severe aortic regurgitation imposes a burden of volume overload on the left ventricle. There is usually an initial phase of compensatory global left ventricular dilatation and cardiac hypertrophy, which eventually progresses to left ventricular systolic dysfunction. Evidence of this should be sought, as it supports a diagnosis of severe regurgitation, although other causes of left ventricular dysfunction may obviously coexist in the same patient. Conversely, in the absence of left ventricular dilatation, aortic regurgitation is unlikely to be severe.

Estimates of left ventricular ejection fraction and M-mode measurement of left ventricular dimensions are essential for selecting asymptomatic patients with severe aortic regurgitation who may benefit from aortic valve replacement.

Assessment of acute aortic regurgitation

In chronic aortic regurgitation compensatory mechanisms allow the left ventricle to adapt to the additional volume of blood, and left ventricular volume increases to maintain a relatively normal end diastolic pressure and normal systolic function. In contrast, in acute severe aortic regurgitation, no adaptation is possible, and left ventricular end diastolic pressure is very elevated. The left ventricle therefore appears to be normal in size, and by certain criteria aortic regurgitation can appear unimpressive, despite devastating haemodynamic effects. In this situation vena contracta width and quantitative echo measures are more reliable.

Causes of aortic regurgitation

Common causes of aortic regurgitation can be divided into those that cause disruption of aortic valve cusp coaptation and those that cause destruction of the aortic valve itself (Table 12.3). The appearance of the aortic valve on two-dimensional echo will often give an indication of the cause, e.g. aortic root dilatation (Fig. 19.4), aortic dissection, bicuspid valve (Fig. 12.12), valve calcification/immobility, flail cusp and vegetation (Fig. 15.5).

Surgery for aortic regurgitation

Acute severe aortic regurgitation requires emergency aortic valve replacement after initial medical stabilisation.

Table 12.3 Causes of aortic regurgitation

Pathology	Echo appearance
Cusp deformity	
Calcific degeneration	Calcified, immobile cusps
Endocarditis	Vegetation, perforation, flail cusp, abscess
Rheumatic heart disease	Calcified, immobile cusps, commissural thickening
Acute rheumatic fever	Thickened immobile cusps
Congenital deformity	Bicuspid, quadricuspid, prolapsing aortic valve
Ventricular septal defect	Displaced aortic root, malaligned ventricular septal defect
Ruptured sinus of Valsalva aneurysm	Dilated sinus, atrial regurgitation jet into right ventricle
Root dilatation	
Aortic root aneurysm	Root dilatation: evidence of underlying cause, e.g. Marfan's syndrome, coarctation, hypertension
Aortic dissection	Dissection flap, false lumen, pericardial effusion, aneurysm

In chronic severe aortic regurgitation the timing of aortic valve replacement depends on the symptoms of the patient and evidence of left ventricular remodelling. Severe left ventricular dysfunction/dilatation may be irreversible and these patients may not benefit from aortic valve replacement. Therefore surgery is considered in symptomatic patients as long as left ventricular function is not severely impaired (ejection fraction >25%) or excessively dilated (end systolic left ventricular diameter of 5.5 cm or less, end diastolic diameter of 7.5 cm or less). In asymptomatic patients with severe chronic aortic regurgitation it is current practice to wait for evidence of progressive left ventricular remodelling before recommending surgery (e.g. systolic left ventricular internal diameter 4.5–5.5 cm, or mild-to-moderate left ventricular impairment (ejection fraction <55%).

As with aortic stenosis, aortic regurgitation of moderate severity or more may warrant aortic valve replacement if coronary artery bypass grafting or other cardiac surgery is already indicated for other reasons.

Congenital abnormalities

Bicuspid aortic valve

Bicuspid aortic valves often remain undetected at birth and may present in adulthood with murmurs and evidence of aortic valve dysfunction. Although the cusps

Figure 12.12

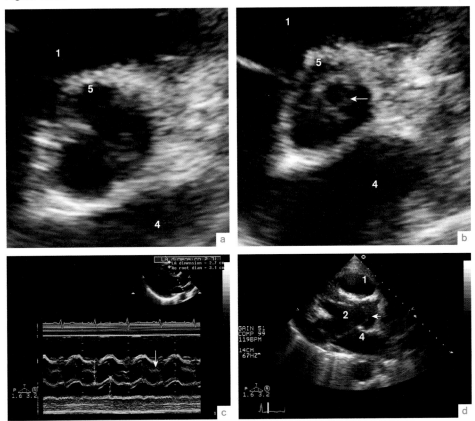

Examples of Bicuspid aortic valves. (a and **b)** Parasternal short axis view at aortic valve level. There is a single closure line from 10 to 4 o'clock. Part of the anterior cusp prolapses (arrow), causing aortic regurgitation. **(c)** M-mode parasternal long axis (PSLAX) view: note the eccentric closure line. **(d)** PSLAX view: during systole the cusps are characteristically domed (arrowhead).

View **On-line** Images

are initially pliable, flow is turbulent and predisposes to premature degeneration. This leads to valve stenosis, regurgitation, or a mixture of both. It may also be associated with aortic root dilatation and aortic coarctation, and these abnormalities should be actively excluded in any patient with a bicuspid aortic valve. Lifelong follow-up is required because of the inevitable progressive valve dysfunction.

The presence of only two cusps is best seen in the PSSAX view (Fig. 12.12a), though the appearance is not always unambiguous. The cusps are often of unequal size and the closure line in PSLAX M-mode is eccentric (Fig. 12.12c). Another feature is systolic 'doming', which arises because the tips are fused together, whilst the bodies of the cusps remain pliable and bend under the pressure of blood flow (Fig. 12.12d).

Sometimes a structurally tricuspid aortic valve has a congenitally fused raphe between two cusps, so the valve is functionally bicuspid (Fig. 12.13).

Figure 12.13

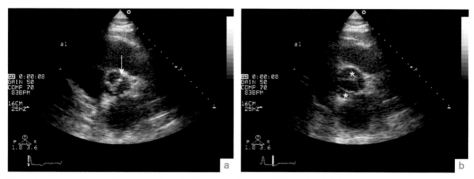

Fused aortic valve raphe. Parasternal short axis views. **(a)** Diastole. **(b)** Systole. The raphe between the right and left coronary cusps is fused (arrow), making this valve functionally bicuspid. This is best appreciated in systole when two cusps are clearly seen (*).

View **On-line** Images

Figure 12.14

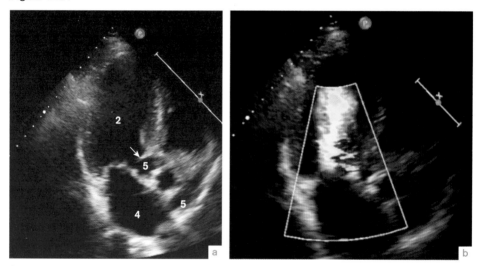

Subvalvular aortic stenosis. Apical three-chamber view. **(a)** A distinct muscular ridge is seen in the left ventricular outflow tract (arrow). The aortic valve is also diseased, and the aortic root is dilated. **(b)** Aortic regurgitation is also evident.

View **On-line** Images

Quadricuspid aortic valve

Rarely the aortic valve may have four separate valve cusps, which can be associated with aortic regurgitation in later life. It may also be associated with other congenital malformations.

Subvalvular aortic stenosis

A variety of congenital abnormalities can cause LVOT narrowing and obstruction. These are usually fibromuscular ridges or membranes extending between the septum and mitral valve annulus, or focal muscular obstruction (Fig. 12.14). The aortic valve itself can be congenitally abnormal: in addition, the turbulent flow across the membrane can damage the aortic valve and often leads to aortic regurgitation.

Although rare, these conditions can present in adulthood and are frequently mistaken for aortic valve stenosis. Careful assessment of the aortic valve and site of obstruction using PW Doppler is required to reach the correct diagnosis.

Supravalvular aortic stenosis

Supravalvular obstruction can be caused by congenital narrowing of the ascending aorta and is commonly seen in Williams' syndrome (Fig. 12.15). Most commonly this occurs at the sinotubular junction or above the coronary sinuses. More rarely it is due to generalised underdevelopment of the aorta.

Figure 12.15

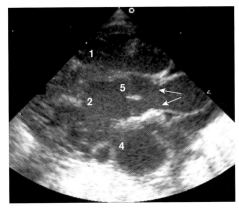

Supravalvular aortic stenosis. Parasternal long axis view. There is an obvious narrowing of the ascending aorta at the sinotubular junction (arrows).

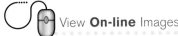
View **On-line** Images

Reporting box

Reporting on aortic stenosis

Summary

- Underlying cause
- Severity

Qualitative data

- Structure of valve: bicuspid, tricuspid, etc.
- Calcification: severity and distribution
- Cusp opening: degree of restriction

(Continued)

Reporting box *Continued*

Quantitative data

- Peak velocity
- Peak instantaneous gradient
- Mean gradient
- Calculated aortic valve area
- Planimetered valve area (transoesophageal echocardiography)

Other findings

- Left ventricular mass
- Left ventricular systolic and diastolic function
- Other valvular disease
- Evidence of sub-/supravalvular obstruction
- Aortic root structure

Reporting box

Reporting on aortic regurgitation

Summary

- Underlying cause
- Severity

Qualitative data

- Structure of valve: bicuspid, tricuspid, etc.
- Aortic root structure
- Calcification: severity and distribution
- Cusp integrity, evidence of vegetations, etc.
- Descending aortic flow reversal

Quantitative data

- Vena contracta width
- Jet width: left ventricular outflow tract ratio
- Pressure half-time/deceleration
- Effective regurgitant orifice area
- Regurgitant fraction/volume

Other findings

- Left ventricular dimensions
- Left ventricular function
- Other valvular disease
- Aortic root diameter

CHAPTER

13

The mitral valve

The normal mitral valve

The mitral valve is a complex structure comprising two valve leaflets and a subvalvular apparatus of chordae and papillary muscles. The leaflets are semicircular in shape and the anterior leaflet is the larger of the two. Each leaflet has three scallops (Fig. 13.1a), or segments. The leaflets attach to a fibrous mitral annulus, which is in continuity with the fibrous rings of the other valves.

The leaflets are intrinsically pliable and rely on the support of the subvalvular structures to prevent leaflet prolapse. The chordae are fibrous strings that attach the leaflets to the anterolateral and posteromedial papillary muscle groups. These arise from the free wall of the left ventricle and attach to both mitral valve leaflets. During systole the papillary muscles contract and brace the leaflets against the high ventricular pressure. The integrity of all components of the mitral valve apparatus is required to maintain proper function.

Echocardiographic appearance

No single echocardiographic view shows the entire mitral valve, so it is essential to examine it carefully from as many views as possible to build up a complete picture. In the parasternal short axis (PSSAX) view the valve is seen *en face* and the segments of the leaflets can be defined, roughly as indicated in Figure 13.1a. The ultrasound beam should be aligned with the leaflet tips to view the valve orifice, and swung cranially to view the leaflets. Directing the beam caudally allows the chordae and papillary muscles to be seen (Fig. 13.1b). In the parasternal long axis (PSLAX) and apical views the anterior and posterior leaflets are seen to protrude in the left ventricle, and the subvalvular apparatus is sometimes identifiable (Fig. 13.1c). Rotation between the apical four-, two- and

Figure 13.1

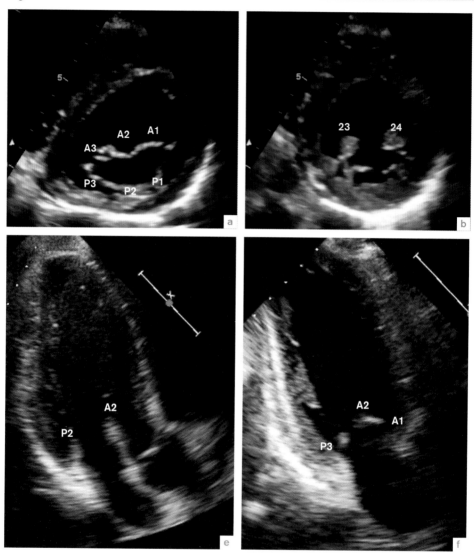

three-chamber (A4C, A2C and A3C) views allows different segments of each leaflet to be scrutinized (Fig. 13.1d–f). A combination of views will allow most of the scallops to be viewed individually.

The mitral leaflets should be thin (no more than 4 mm), pliable and non-calcified. In diastole they open widely into the left ventricle in a biphasic manner. The first phase occurs as diastole begins, and this is followed by partial recoil of the leaflets. As atrial contraction occurs in late diastole the leaflets are forced apart again, until final closure occurs with the onset of systole. This can be appreciated by scrolling through a recording of a mitral valve in slow motion. M-mode from the PSLAX aligned with the leaflet tips will also demonstrate this pattern (Fig. 13.1g).

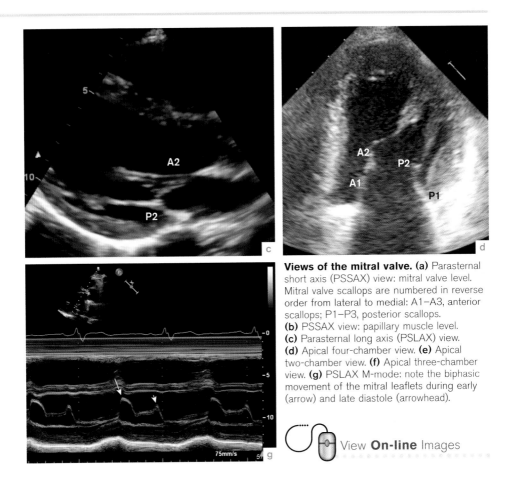

Views of the mitral valve. (a) Parasternal short axis (PSSAX) view: mitral valve level. Mitral valve scallops are numbered in reverse order from lateral to medial: A1–A3, anterior scallops; P1–P3, posterior scallops. **(b)** PSSAX view: papillary muscle level. **(c)** Parasternal long axis (PSLAX) view. **(d)** Apical four-chamber view. **(e)** Apical two-chamber view. **(f)** Apical three-chamber view. **(g)** PSLAX M-mode: note the biphasic movement of the mitral leaflets during early (arrow) and late diastole (arrowhead).

View **On-line** Images

The mitral annulus diameter should be measured from the A4C view at end diastole, and should be less than 3.4 cm.

Doppler examination

Transmitral blood flow should be routinely interrogated from the A4C view using pulse wave (PW) Doppler with the sample volume positioned at the tip of the mitral valve leaflets. Normal diastolic flow in sinus rhythm is biphasic with an early (E) wave, and a later atrial (A) wave (Fig. 13.2). Normal values for peak velocities are given in Table 13.1. Inaccurate placement of the sample volume can alter the absolute values of the peak E and A wave velocity, but will not usually affect the ratio. The pattern of transmitral flow is informative about mitral valve function, left atrial pressure and left ventricular diastolic function (Chapter 5). It is common to detect a trivial amount of mitral regurgitation by colour flow mapping (CFM) or spectral Doppler.

Figure 13.2

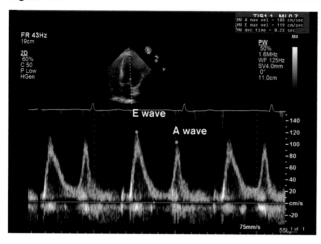

Transmitral pulse wave Doppler. The sample volume is placed at the mitral valve leaflet tips. The E and A wave peak velocities and E wave deceleration time are indicated.

Table 13.1 Normal values for transmitral flow

	<50 years	>50 years
E wave peak velocity (cm/s)	72 ± 14	62 ± 14
A wave peak velocity (cm/s)	40 ± 10	59 ± 14
E:A ratio	1.9 ± 0.6	1.1 ± 0.3
Deceleration time (ms)	179 ± 20	210 ± 36

Values are mean ± SD.

The pattern of blood flow from the pulmonary veins into the left atrium is affected by mitral valve disease and should be routinely interrogated. This is discussed in more detail in later sections.

Diseases of the mitral valve

Like any valve, the mitral valve is susceptible to a wide variety of pathologies. In this section pathologies that are relatively specific to the mitral valve will be discussed in more detail. Sections on endocarditis (Chapter 15), ischaemic and functional mitral regurgitation (Chapter 8) and cardiomyopathy (Chapter 9) should also be consulted.

Mitral annular calcification

This is a degenerative process that is usually an incidental finding. It is more common in elderly patients and those with renal insufficiency. The annular ring becomes calcified, and this process may extend to the mitral valve leaflets themselves (Fig. 13.3). This makes the ring and leaflets highly echogenic and can mimic

Figure 13.3

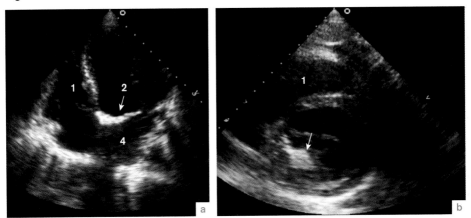

Mitral annular calcification. (a) Apical four-chamber view. Severe mitral annular calcification localised to the anterior mitral annulus, extending to the anterior mitral leaflet. Note the very bright appearance of the calcium deposits. **(b)** Parasternal short axis view. Nodular mitral annular calcification, confined to the posterior mitral annulus.

View **On-line** Images

rheumatic valve disease. The calcification process can be diffuse or localised. In the majority of cases it has no functional consequences, but very extensive calcification can lead to restricted leaflet movement and may cause regurgitation or, very rarely, stenosis.

Rheumatic mitral valve disease (RMVD)

Rheumatic fever is an inflammatory condition triggered by group A streptococcal pharyngeal infection: it is rare in the Western world, but is a significant healthcare problem in developing countries.

It has two phases: in the acute phase there is systemic inflammation affecting many organs, including the valves, endocardium, myocardium and pericardium of the heart. Any valve can be affected, but the mitral and aortic valves are particularly prone to rheumatic damage. In the acute phase mitral valve leaflets and chordae may be inflamed, causing thickening, sometimes with evidence of valve nodules, chordal elongation and, rarely, rupture.

Chronic/recurrent inflammation can result in severe valvular damage after 10 years or more. Characteristically there is fusion of the commissures between the leaflets, and chordal retraction, so that the valve does not open fully, but the leaflets remain pliable. On transthoracic echocardiography there is a 'hockey stick' appearance to the anterior mitral valve leaflet in which the mitral valve tips appear fused together, whilst the remainder of the leaflets bulge into the left ventricle during diastole, due to raised left atrial pressure (Fig. 13.4). Eventually, calcification occurs, and the leaflets/chordae become thickened, immobile and echo-bright (Fig. 13.5). This process may lead to valve stenosis, regurgitation or a mixture of both. The assessment of rheumatic mitral stenosis will be discussed later in this chapter.

Figure 13.4

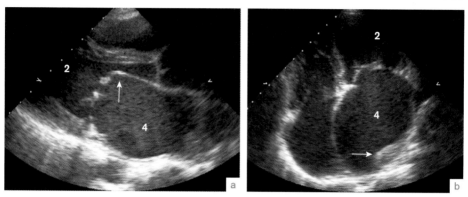

Rheumatic mitral valve disease. (a) Parasternal long axis view. The classic 'hockey stick' appearance of the anterior mitral valve leaflet (arrow), due to thickening and restriction of the leaflet tips. There is minimal calcification. Note spontaneous echo contrast within the left atrium. **(b)** Apical four-chamber view. The left atrium is very dilated and thrombus is evident (arrow).

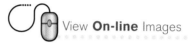 View **On-line** Images

Figure 13.5

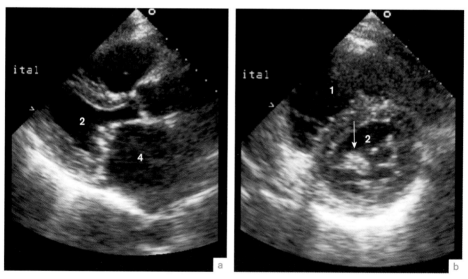

Rheumatic mitral valve disease. (a) Parasternal long axis view: note the severe calcification of the leaflet tips and chordae. **(b)** Parasternal short axis view: in this view severe calcification of the medial commissure is well seen (arrow).

View **On-line** Images

Mitral valve prolapse

This condition is characterised by myxomatous degeneration of the mitral valve leaflets, which leads to leaflet thickening, redundancy and floppiness. Leaflets prolapse across the plane of the mitral annulus during systole and fail to coapt properly, leading to regurgitation. Sometimes mitral valve prolapse (MVP) is a manifestation of an underlying syndrome such as collagen disorders (Ehlers–Danlos, osteogenesis imperfecta) or Marfan's syndrome.

The precise echocardiographic criteria for diagnosing MVP are:

1. Systolic displacement of one or both leaflets behind the plane of the annulus in the PSLAX view (Fig. 13.6).
2. Movement of the point of apposition behind the plane of the annulus in the A4C view (Fig. 13.7).

Leaflet thickness exceeding 5 mm on fundamental imaging (i.e. not using tissue harmonics) is also highly supportive evidence for MVP (Figs 13.6 and 13.7). The posterior mitral valve leaflet, particularly the P2 segment, is most commonly affected. When only one leaflet prolapses, the jet of regurgitant blood is eccentric, and is directed towards the normal leaflet (Fig. 13.7). If both prolapse equally, the jet is central. Additional findings include evidence of annular dilatation, chordal redundancy, chordal rupture and flail segments (Fig. 13.8).

Cases of MVP usually require echocardiographic follow-up, depending on the severity of valve dysfunction, as mitral valve surgery may become necessary. Increasingly, techniques to repair prolapsing valves can avoid the need for mitral valve replacement, and this may be considered at an earlier stage in the course of disease than valve replacement. Suitability for repair is best assessed using trans-oesophageal echocardiography (TOE).

Figure 13.6

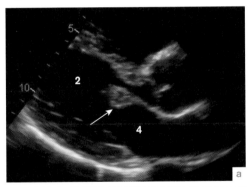

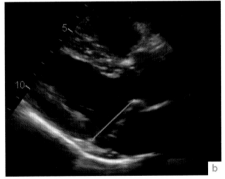

Mitral valve prolapse. Parasternal long axis view. **(a)** End diastole. **(b)** End systole. **(c)** Early systole. The anterior mitral valve leaflet is very thickened and 'fleshy' (arrow). During systole there is prolapse behind the plane of the mitral annulus (red line). A very eccentric, posteriorly directed jet of mitral regurgitation is seen.

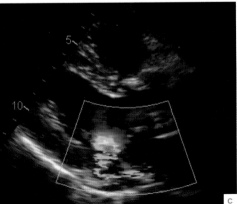

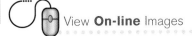

View **On-line** Images

Figure 13.7

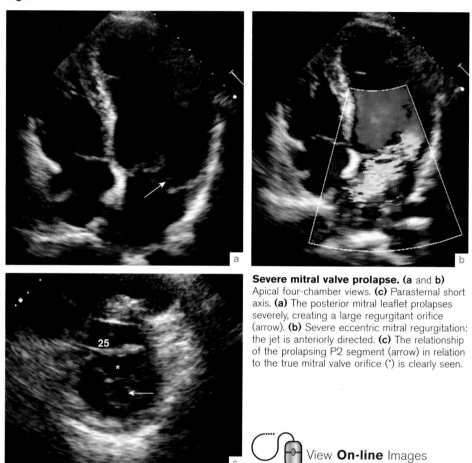

Severe mitral valve prolapse. (a and **b)** Apical four-chamber views. **(c)** Parasternal short axis. **(a)** The posterior mitral leaflet prolapses severely, creating a large regurgitant orifice (arrow). **(b)** Severe eccentric mitral regurgitation: the jet is anteriorly directed. **(c)** The relationship of the prolapsing P2 segment (arrow) in relation to the true mitral valve orifice (*) is clearly seen.

View **On-line** Images

Assessing severity of mitral regurgitation

Mitral regurgitation occurs when blood leaks through the mitral valve during left ventricular contraction. A small amount of regurgitation is commonly seen in healthy individuals who have no demonstrable valvular abnormality, and this is considered to be physiological.

Detection

Mitral regurgitation can be detected easily using CFM, and this is best appreciated from the apical views, where the regurgitant flow is directly away from the probe, and coloured blue. Evidence of mitral regurgitation can also be detected using spectral Doppler. When mitral regurgitation is detected you should try to answer three important questions: is it severe, what is the cause, and is there evidence of cardiac decompensation?

Figure 13.8

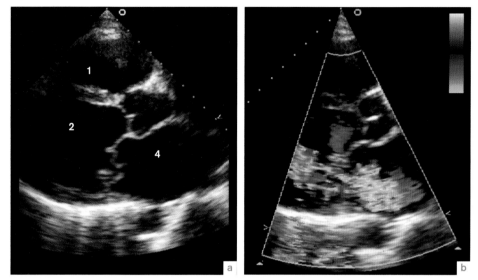

Flail mitral valve secondary to chordal rupture. Parasternal long axis views. **(a)** There is obvious bileaflet prolapse with failure of coaptation. The leaflet tips are flail, and fragments of chord can be seen to move independently of the leaflets. Note also the compensatory tachycardia. **(b)** Severe mitral regurgitation.

View **On-line** Images

How severe is the mitral regurgitation?

The severity of mitral regurgitation is simply determined by the volume of blood leaking through the valve into the left atrium. As discussed in Chapter 11, this cannot be measured directly by echocardiographic techniques, so a variety of other measures are used instead. It is absolutely critical to realise that no single measurement can be relied on to define the severity of regurgitation, so a complete assessment requires many different parameters to be taken into account.

A wide variety of techniques can be used, and emphasis should be given to specific parameters that are considered most reliable, whilst less reliable ones can be used as supportive evidence. This hierarchical approach is summarised in Figure 13.9, whilst Table 13.2 gives generally accepted values for each parameter.

Specific measures

Structural signs

In certain situations the structural appearance of the mitral valve should alert you to the possibility of severe regurgitation. This particularly applies to flail leaflets and papillary muscle rupture, which can cause acute catastrophic regurgitation.

A flail mitral leaflet usually occurs as a complication of MVP (Fig. 13.8) or endocarditis, due to rupture of a chord or degeneration of the leaflet itself. The appearance depends on the exact cause: sometimes the leaflet can be seen to be abnormally mobile, prolapsing completely into the left atrium during systole and flopping back into the left ventricle in diastole. Ruptured chordae may also be

Figure 13.9

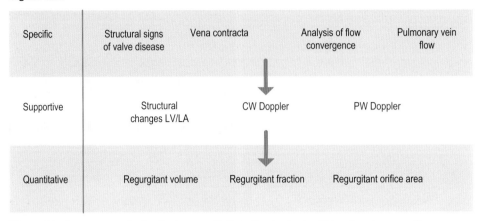

Hierarchical assessment of mitral regurgitation. Emphasis should be placed on specific parameters. Supportive parameters should be given less weight in decision making. Further discrimination can be sought from quantitative measures, if the operator has experience in this. LV, left ventricle; LA, left atrium; CW, continuous wave; PW, pulse wave.

Table 13.2 Grading mitral regurgitation (MR)

Parameter	Mild MR	Severe MR
Specific		
Vena contracta diameter (cm)	<0.3	≥0.7
PISA lite radius* (cm)	<0.4	≥1.0
Pulmonary vein flow	Normal	Systolic flow reversal
Supportive		
LV dilatation	Not present	Usually present
Pulmonary hypertension	Not present	Often present
CW Doppler	Not dense	Dense, triangular
PW Doppler	Can be E<A wave	Never E<A wave
Quantitative		
Regurgitant orifice area (cm²)	<0.2	≥0.4
Regurgitant volume (ml/beat)	<30	≥60
Regurgitant fraction (%)	<30	≥50

PISA, proximal isovelocity surface area; LV, left ventricular; CW, continuous wave; PW, pulse wave.
*Aliasing velocity set to 40 cm/s.

visible, either attached to the leaflet and independently mobile like a vegetation, or wafting freely in the left ventricle. However, because multiple chordae are attached to each leaflet it is possible for just one portion to become flail, whilst the rest remains relatively normal. This emphasises the importance of assessing all segments of the valve from different angles; otherwise, important structural clues will be missed.

Papillary muscle rupture most commonly occurs after myocardial infarction (Fig. 8.6), but can also complicate endocarditis. Again, partial rupture may not be very obvious and the whole valve needs to be studied carefully.

Vena contracta width

The vena contracta is the narrowest portion of the regurgitant jet, just after the orifice, as viewed by CFM Doppler (Fig. 13.10). Vena contracta width correlates with the width of the regurgitant orifice and therefore regurgitation severity. It is not influenced by CFM gain settings as much as jet length/area, but the width can vary during systole, and the widest vena contracta should be measured. In general, the best estimates are obtained from the PSLAX view, whilst the A2C view tends to overestimate the severity of mitral regurgitation. The image should be magnified if possible to minimise measurement errors.

Mild mitral regurgitation is present if the vena contracta diameter is less than 3 mm, whilst a diameter ≥7 mm is indicative of severe regurgitation.

PISA lite

Proximal isovelocity surface area (PISA) is a method of estimating effective regurgitant orifice area (EROA) by analysing the flow convergence zone of a regurgitant

Figure 13.10

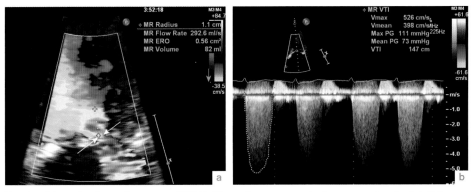

Proximal isovelocity surface area (PISA) lite and assessment of vena contracta. (a) Colour flow mapping Doppler: measurement of radius and vena contracta width. **(b)** Spectral Doppler: measurement of velocity time integral.
PISA: The colour scale baseline has been adjusted downwards (green arrow) so that the lower limit is approximately 40 cm/s. This creates an abrupt transition between blue and yellow, allowing the PISA radius to be measured as demonstrated. Under these settings PISA lite can be applied: the radius is >1.0 cm, indicating severe mitral regurgitation. Effective regurgitant orifice area (EROA) has been calculated as 0.56 cm^2.
Regurgitant volume: this can be estimated by measuring the mitral regurgitant velocity time integral and EROA.
Vena contracta: this is indicated by the arrows, as the jet passes through the valve orifice.

jet, as described in Chapter 11. PISA lite is a simplification of this calculation applied specifically to mitral regurgitation. It cannot be applied to other valves.

It is based on the assumption that the peak velocity of the mitral regurgitation jet (V_{max}) is approximately 500 cm/s: in most cases this is a reasonable assumption because the left ventricular pressure greatly exceeds left atrial pressure (100 mmHg gradient = 500 cm/s velocity). If the aliasing velocity of the CFM Doppler (V_a) is set to 40 cm/s the PISA equation can be simplified to:

$$EROA = \frac{2\pi r^2 \times V_a}{V_{max}}$$

$$EROA = \frac{2 \times 3.142 \times r^2 \times 40}{500}$$

$$EROA = \frac{r^2}{2}$$

This means that EROA can be estimated simply by measuring the radius of the PISA shell, at an aliasing velocity of 40 cm/s. In fact, the situation can be simplified even further since severe regurgitation (EROA >0.4 cm^2) equates to a PISA lite radius (r) of 1.0 cm or more.

In practical terms PISA lite requires a good-quality magnified image of the flow convergence zone. The aliasing velocity is adjusted to 40 cm/s to maximise the colour contrast at the PISA: in the A4C view the baseline should be shifted downwards (in the direction of the regurgitant jet) so that the lower-range aliasing velocity is set to approximately 40 cm/s: this gives a blue–yellow colour scale. The radius of the PISA shell is then measured from the colour interface of the aliasing shell to the regurgitant orifice. If this is 1.0 cm or greater, mitral regurgitation is severe (Fig. 13.10).

Pulmonary vein flow

Pulmonary vein flow into the left atrium normally occurs in both systole and diastole, with systolic flow predominating. In the presence of severe mitral regurgitation forward flow into the left atrium may be blunted or even reversed during systole (Fig. 13.11) due to raised left atrial pressure. Indeed, regurgitant jets can sometimes be seen to extend far back into the pulmonary veins on CFM Doppler, indicating actual reversal of flow.

To assess pulmonary vein flow you need to obtain a good-quality A4C view. Use CFM Doppler with a high gain setting to identify the right inferior or superior pulmonary vein, near the interatrial septum. Place the PW sample volume 1 cm within the vein and adjust the velocity scale and picture depth to ensure aliasing is avoided. Practice is required to perform and interpret this technique correctly.

Supportive measurements

Structural signs

In chronic severe mitral regurgitation cardiac output can only be maintained if the stroke volume of the heart increases, and this is achieved over months or years by a combination of left ventricular dilatation and sometimes increased contractility. Ultimately, these compensatory mechanisms cannot be sustained indefinitely, and

Figure 13.11

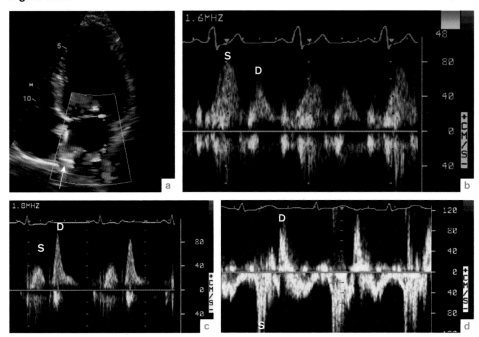

Pulmonary vein flow. (a) Apical four-chamber view: the pulse wave sample volume is placed in the right inferior pulmonary vein guided by colour flow mapping Doppler (arrow). **(b)** Normal pulmonary vein flow. The systolic wave (S) is bigger than the diastolic wave (D). **(c)** Blunted systolic forward flow (S<D). **(d)** Systolic flow reversal.

View **On-line** Images

uncorrected severe mitral regurgitation eventually leads to irreversible left ventricular dilatation and failure.

It is important to note that severe mitral regurgitation can 'flatter' the appearance of left ventricular function because a significant volume of blood is ejected into the left atrium, which is low-pressure and highly compliant. Therefore measurements of left ventricular ejection fraction (EF) will be augmented, and this should be taken into account: accordingly, in the presence of significant mitral regurgitation, normal EF is greater than 60%.

Leakage of a high-pressure jet of blood into the left atrium increases left atrial pressure, which in turn creates a build-up of pressure in the pulmonary veins, and eventually the pulmonary arteries. This backlog can cause left atrial enlargement, pulmonary hypertension, right heart failure and tricuspid regurgitation. Identification of these features provides confirmatory evidence of the severity of mitral regurgitation, assuming other potential causes are not present.

Continuous wave Doppler of mitral regurgitant jet

The Doppler signal is really just a graphical representation of the speed of red blood cell flow against time. The appearance of this depends on the pattern of blood flow: regurgitation through an abnormal valve is usually turbulent, rather than laminar, with blood cells travelling in many different directions at different speeds, and so the Doppler signal is 'filled in'. If there is severe regurgitation, more red blood cells are present in the jet, making the Doppler signal appear dense. This can be assessed by aligning a continuous wave Doppler cursor through the vena contracta of the mitral regurgitation jet, visualised on CFM from an apical view (Fig. 13.12). The density of the regurgitant jet is compared to that of the forward flow in diastole. The duration of regurgitation can also be used as a guide to severity: moderate-to-severe mitral regurgitation usually lasts for the whole of systole. When mitral regurgitation is severe the contour of the Doppler spectrum may be triangular, with an early systolic peak, rather than the typical rounded appearance (Fig. 13.12).

The obvious disadvantage of this technique is that it is very subjective. In addition, poor alignment with the mitral regurgitation jet is prone to lead to underestimation, especially if it is eccentric, or there are multiple jets.

Pulse wave Doppler
Transmitral forward flow should be assessed using PW Doppler with the sample volume at the tips of the mitral valve leaflets. In severe mitral regurgitation (in the absence of mitral stenosis) there is often dominant early left ventricular filling due

Figure 13.12

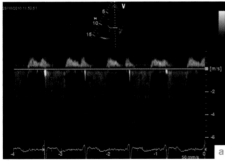

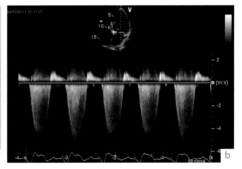

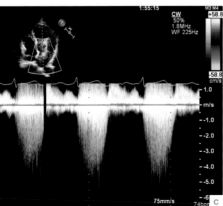

Continuous wave Doppler assessment of mitral regurgitation. (a) Mild mitral regurgitation. **(b)** Moderate mitral regurgitation. **(c)** Severe mitral regurgitation.

to raised left atrial pressure, which is reflected by a dominant E wave peak velocity (>120 cm/s) compared to the A wave. Put another way, A wave dominance suggests that mitral regurgitation is not severe.

Other measures

Jet area/length

A large volume of regurgitation is suggested by a wide jet that reaches far back into the left atrium. However, jet width, area and length are deemed unreliable due to dependence on gain settings. Furthermore, eccentric jets that hit the atrial wall are underestimated by about 40% due to physical restriction of flow and limited 'recruitment' of adjacent blood. This is known as the Coanda effect.

Quantitative estimates of mitral regurgitant severity

Regurgitant volume and regurgitant fraction

Quantitative techniques for estimating regurgitant volume and regurgitant fraction can be made by determining the stroke volumes of the left and right ventricles. The methodology of this is discussed in Chapter 11.

A regurgitant volume of more than 60 ml or regurgitant fraction greater than 50% of left ventricular inflow volume is considered severe.

PISA

Calculation of EROA using PISA is covered in Chapter 11. An EROA of 0.4 cm^2 or greater is considered indicative of severe mitral regurgitation, whilst less than 0.2 cm^2 suggests mild regurgitation.

Acute mitral regurgitation

Acute severe mitral regurgitation requires special consideration as the physiology and echocardiographic features differ markedly from chronic mitral regurgitation. It occurs in conditions that cause flail leaflets, chordal rupture or papillary rupture, such as MVP, endocarditis and myocardial infarction.

Sudden mitral valve incompetence usually causes acute pulmonary oedema/cardiogenic shock, because a large component of the left ventricular stroke volume is ejected into the left atrium. Left atrial pressure is extremely high because atrial compliance (distensibility) is low and insufficient time has elapsed for compensatory dilatation. Equally, left ventricular size is usually normal, and left ventricular function often appears vigorous.

Under these conditions the basic criteria for assessing mitral regurgitation severity are usually unreliable, and it is easy to underestimate the severity (Fig. 8.6). Specific methods such as vena contracta width and PISA should be used. In addition, evidence of significant structural mitral valve disease (e.g. flail leaflet) should alert you to the possibility of severe mitral regurgitation.

What is the cause?

Mitral regurgitation can be caused by problems with any part of the mitral apparatus. The basic mechanisms can be divided into those that affect the integrity of the leaflets, the papillary/chordal apparatus, the annulus or any combination. Possible causes are listed in Table 13.3.

A diagnosis of 'mitral regurgitation' is incomplete unless an underlying explanation is identified. This is vital because it determines further treatment options, such as suitability for mitral valve replacement/repair, need for antibiotic treatment, heart failure therapy, and so on.

Table 13.3 Causes and mechanisms of mitral regurgitation

Cause	Mechanism
Functional	Annular dilatation/papillary displacement secondary to heart failure
Ischaemic heart disease	Papillary muscle rupture
	Papillary muscle dysfunction
	Annular dilatation/papillary displacement secondary to heart failure
Mitral valve prolapse	Floppy leaflet
	Flail leaflet
	Chordal rupture
Rheumatic	Leaflet fibrosis/calcification
	Chordal fibrosis/calcification
Infective endocarditis	Leaflet destruction
	Chordal rupture
HOCM	Systolic anterior motion of the mitral valve
	Papillary abnormalities
Miscellaneous	
Amyloid	Leaflet/chordal thickening
Endomyocardial fibrosis	Leaflet/chordal thickening
SLE	Leaflet/chordal thickening
Marantic endocarditis	Leaflet/chordal thickening
Congenital	
Cleft leaflet	Defective leaflet
Endocardial cushion defect	Defective leaflet
Double orifice mitral valve	Defective leaflet
Parachute mitral valve	Papillary abnormality

HOCM, hypertrophic obstructive cardiomyopathy; SLE, systemic lupus erythematosus.

The appearance of the mitral valve will often give a major clue about the underlying cause. You should look for evidence of valve thickening, calcification, prolapse, vegetation, flail segment, ruptured chordae, papillary dysfunction/rupture and annular dilatation. If the valve is structurally normal, with evidence of left ventricular dilatation/dysfunction, functional regurgitation may be the cause.

Surgery for mitral regurgitation

Echo practitioners may not be directly involved in deciding on the necessity of mitral valve surgery, but it is important to have an appreciation of the criteria, so that reports are comprehensive and accurate.

In general, acute severe mitral regurgitation with haemodynamic compromise requires emergency surgery to repair or replace the valve. Echocardiography is essential for the detection and assessment of the underlying cause, and perioperative TOE is required to guide surgery.

In chronic severe mitral regurgitation, surgery is usually considered for primary mitral valve disease, such as MVP and RMVD, rather than secondary causes such as functional mitral regurgitation. In general the best results are obtained if the mitral valve can be repaired, rather than replaced, and before left ventricular dysfunction/pulmonary hypertension has developed: if surgery is left too late, left ventricular dysfunction may be irreversible. Optimal timing of surgery therefore depends on symptoms, likelihood of valve repair and evidence of cardiac decompensation.

Surgery is indicated in symptomatic patients with severe mitral regurgitation as long as left ventricular function is preserved. Surgery may not be desirable if left ventricular function is severely impaired or dilated (EF <30% and systolic left ventricular internal diameter (LVIDs) >55 mm), though each case has to be considered on its individual merits.

In asymptomatic patients with severe mitral regurgitation, evidence of progressive compensatory change in left ventricular diameter is usually sought before recommending surgery, unless mitral repair is likely, or decompensation is already apparent (EF <60%, LVIDs >45 mm, pulmonary artery systolic pressure >50 mmHg).

It is common practice to confirm mitral regurgitation severity by TOE prior to surgery. This gives detailed images of all the mitral valve components, as well as allowing an assessment of the likelihood of surgical repair versus replacement in cases of MVP.

Mitral stenosis

The normal mitral valve area (MVA) in an average adult is around 4–6 cm², but reduction to less than 2.0 cm² indicates valve stenosis. Severe stenosis occurs when the orifice area is reduced to <1 cm². The predominant cause is rheumatic mitral disease, though rarer causes include mitral annular calcification, systemic lupus erythematosus, carcinoid syndrome, congenital mitral stenosis, amyloidosis and disorders of glycolipid metabolism. In all cases the mitral valve leaflets become thickened and immobile, obstructing blood flow between the left atrium and left ventricle.

The natural history and echocardiographic features of chronic rheumatic mitral stenosis are described above (Figs 13.4 and 13.5).

Assessing the severity of mitral stenosis

The severity of mitral stenosis reflects the reduction in MVA, and this can be estimated in three ways. In general more than one method should be used to confirm the findings of another.

Planimetry

This involves imaging the mitral valve in the PSSAX view at the leaflet tips, so that the orifice area can be measured directly by tracing with a cursor (Fig. 13.13). Measurement is made in early diastole when valve opening should be maximal. To be accurate the probe must be completely in line with the plane of the valve at the leaflet tips. It is unreliable if alignment is suboptimal, if there is significant tip calcification or previous mitral valve surgery. Three-dimensional echo has significant advantages over conventional two-dimensional echo in this respect. Values for grading the severity of mitral stenosis are given in Table 13.4.

Figure 13.13

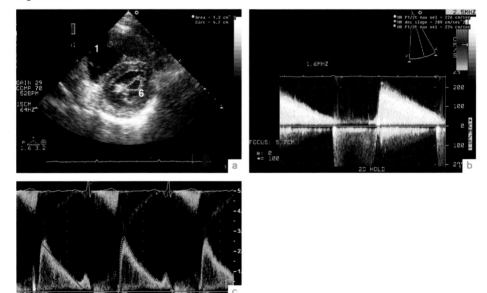

Assessment of mitral stenosis severity.
Planimetry. (a) The mitral valve orifice is visualised in the parasternal short axis view at the level of the mitral valve tips. The circumference of the orifice is traced to obtain an estimate of the area.
Pressure half-time. (b) Pulse wave Doppler is used to interrogate mitral valve inflow at the mitral valve tips. The E wave deceleration is traced as shown to obtain the pressure half-time. **(c)** If the Doppler spectrum has a 'ski slope' pattern, with an early steep deceleration phase followed by a slower phase, the pressure half-time should be measured as shown (red line).
Mean gradient. (c) The pulse wave inflow spectrum is traced as shown to obtain the velocity time integral, from which the mean gradient is automatically calculated.

Table 13.4 Grading mitral stenosis

	Mild	Moderate	Severe
Mitral valve area (cm²)	1.6–2.0	1.0–1.5	<1.0
Pressure half-time (ms)	71–139	140–219	≥220
Mean gradient (mmHg)	<5	6–10	>10

Pressure half-time method

Mitral stenosis causes a pressure gradient between the left atrium and left ventricle in early diastole. If the stenosis is severe, the pressure gradient is sustained, whereas in a mild stenosis pressure declines more rapidly. Since the velocity of blood reflects the pressure gradient (Chapter 11), the rate of decline in velocity across the mitral valve provides information about the MVA. Rather than measuring the pressure gradient, the time taken for the pressure to drop to 50% is measured using continuous wave Doppler. This is known as the pressure half-time, and is not the same as a 50% drop in velocity. Studies in patients have shown that the following equation can be used to estimate MVA reliably:

$$MVA\ (cm^2) = \frac{220}{Pressure\ half\text{-}time\ (ms)}$$

Therefore, a pressure half-time of >220 ms suggests severe stenosis, 140–220 ms suggests moderate stenosis and 71–139 ms is considered mild (Table 13.4).

To measure the pressure half-time, use PW Doppler at the tips of the mitral valve leaflets from the A4C view (Fig. 13.13). This is most accurate if the PW sweep speed is set at 100 mm/s, so that the deceleration slope is easily visualised. Trace the slope of the E wave from the peak to the nadir: most echo machines will automatically calculate the MVA from the pressure half-time.

It is important to be aware of potential limitations of this method. Problems can arise if the Doppler spectrum is not clearly defined, or if deceleration is non-linear, making it difficult to know where exactly to measure. If possible, select a beat with linear E wave deceleration, or else measure the deceleration just after the peak of the slope (Fig. 13.13c). Care should be taken to position the PW sample volume to obtain only the mitral inflow signal, because aortic regurgitant jets can be interrogated by accident.

The method is also less reliable if the heart rate is greater than 100 bpm, as the A wave may obscure the deceleration slope completely. Of course in atrial fibrillation the average of 3–5 beats should be measured.

Mean pressure gradient

Using PW Doppler it is possible to estimate the mean pressure gradient across the stenotic mitral valve by tracing the Doppler spectrum, as shown in Figure 13.13c. Severe stenosis is suggested by a gradient >10 mmHg, moderate 6–10 mmHg and mild <5 mmHg (Table 13.4).

Complications of mitral stenosis

In addition to assessing the severity of stenosis, you should look for complications. Specifically, this should include assessment of:

1. left atrial dimensions
2. presence of thrombus in the left atrial appendage or spontaneous echo contrast (Fig. 13.4)
3. pulmonary artery pressure from tricuspid regurgitation peak velocity
4. right ventricular function
5. evidence of other rheumatic valve lesions.

Surgery for mitral stenosis

Symptomatic patients with an MVA <1.5 cm^2 may be candidates for some form of percutaneous or surgical intervention to the mitral valve. Percutaneous balloon valvuloplasty is feasible as long as there is minimal calcification, no more than mild mitral regurgitation and no evidence of left atrial thrombus on TOE. Surgical valvotomy is sometimes performed in similar cases. In cases where the valve is very degenerate, mitral valve replacement is the only option.

Reporting box

Reporting on mitral regurgitation

Summary

- Severity
- Underlying pathology (e.g. prolapse)
- Mechanism (e.g. flail P2 segment)

Qualitative data

- Leaflet mobility, e.g. normal, prolapse, restriction
- Leaflet thickness and calcification
- Leaflet integrity, e.g. flail leaflet, vegetations, perforation
- Structure of subvalvular apparatus and annulus, e.g. thickening, rupture
- Jet characteristics: central, eccentric, wall impinging, posterior extent

Quantitative data

- Vena contracta
- Proximal isovelocity surface area (PISA) lite radius
- Effective regurgitant orifice area
- Regurgitant fraction/volume

Other

- Left ventricular dimensions and ejection function
- Right ventricular dimensions and function
- Left atrial size
- Pulmonary artery pressure
- Other valvular lesions

Reporting box

Reporting on mitral stenosis

Summary

- Underlying cause
- Severity

Qualitative data

- Valve structure
- Leaflet function: mobility
- Subvalvular structure and function
- Calcification: severity and distribution

Quantitative data

- Pressure half-time
- Mean gradient
- Planimetered valve area

Other

- Pulmonary artery pressure
- Left atrial dimensions
- Other valvular disease

The right heart valves

The normal tricuspid and pulmonary valves

The tricuspid and pulmonary valves more or less mirror the structure, function and physiology of the mitral and aortic valves. Therefore many of the principles of valve assessment that have been learned in previous chapters can be applied to the right heart valves.

The tricuspid valve is situated between the right atrium and the right ventricle and prevents regurgitation of blood into the right atrium during right ventricular systole. There are three major differences compared to the mitral valve. First, the most obvious difference is that the tricuspid valve has three leaflets. Secondly, it is displaced slightly towards the ventricular apex. Finally, the papillary muscles attach to the interventricular septum rather than the free wall.

The pulmonary valve is located at the junction between the right ventricular outflow tract (RVOT) and main pulmonary artery. It has three fibrous cusps, and prevents regurgitation back into the right ventricle.

Echocardiographic appearance

The best views for the tricuspid valve include parasternal long axis (PSLAX) with caudal tilt (right ventricular inflow), parasternal short axis (PSSAX: aortic level), apical four-chamber (A4C) and subcostal views (Fig. 14.1). The valve leaflets should be thin, pliable and non-calcified. There are anterior, posterior and septal leaflets: the septal leaflet is the smallest and least mobile. Although the valve leaflets are usually well seen, the subvalvular apparatus is often less well delineated. The tricuspid annular diameter can be assessed from the A4C view and is <3.8 cm in adults.

Figure 14.1

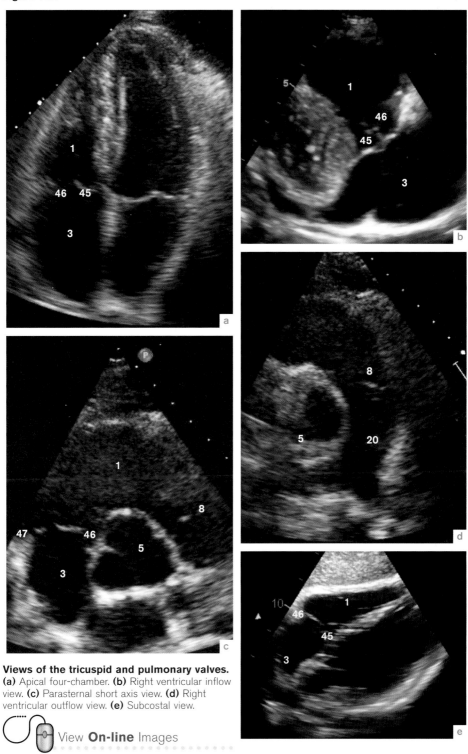

Views of the tricuspid and pulmonary valves.
(a) Apical four-chamber. (b) Right ventricular inflow
view. (c) Parasternal short axis view. (d) Right
ventricular outflow view. (e) Subcostal view.

View **On-line** Images

The pulmonary valve is often poorly visualised on transthoracic echocardiography, but the best views are PSLAX view, with cranial tilt, PSSAX and subcostal short axis views at the aortic level (Figs 14.1b and c). It can be seen that the pulmonary valve lies anteriorly and is roughly perpendicular to the aortic valve. Cusps should be less than 2 mm thick and non-calcified. In some of these views the main pulmonary artery and branches can also be visualised.

Doppler examination

Transtricuspid blood flow mirrors transmitral flow and is best assessed in the A4C view with pulse wave (PW) Doppler positioned at the tips of the tricuspid valve. There is an early diastolic passive phase and a late active phase due to right atrial contraction. Normal values for tricuspid flow are age-dependent, and are roughly 20–30% lower than those across the mitral valve (Appendix 1). Respiratory variation in E wave peak velocity can be as much as 40% in normal subjects. In day-to-day practice detailed analysis of right ventricular diastolic filling is rarely required, the main exception being when pericardial tamponade is suspected.

The main focus of a routine Doppler examination of the tricuspid valve is directed towards the detection and quantification of tricuspid regurgitation, which in turn allows the estimation of pulmonary artery pressure. A trace of tricuspid regurgitation can be detected on colour flow mapping (CFM) or spectral Doppler in the majority of subjects (Fig. 14.2a).

Figure 14.2

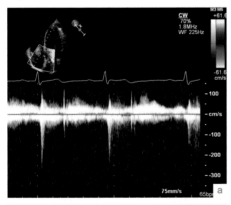
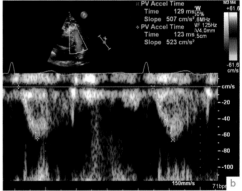
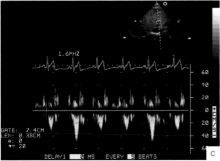

Spectral Doppler. (a) Continuous wave Doppler across the tricuspid valve: linear opening and closing spectra can be seen. There is no detectable tricuspid regurgitation. **(b)** Continuous wave Doppler across the pulmonary valve: forward flow is almost laminar and peak velocity is around 0.7 m/s. Measurement of the pulmonary acceleration time is demonstrated. **(c)** Hepatic vein pulse wave Doppler: note that systolic forward flow (S) is much greater than diastolic flow (D). There is marked respiratory variation in flow velocities.

Flow across the pulmonary valve can be assessed from the PSSAX/right ventricular outflow views using PW or continuous wave (CW) Doppler. Normal peak velocity is between 0.6 and 0.9 m/s (Fig. 14.2b). Trivial pulmonary regurgitation is commonly detectable in normal subjects. Pulmonary acceleration time is useful for estimating pulmonary artery pressure (see below).

Blood flow into the right atrium from the vena cavae is affected by right heart disease and provides important information about right heart function. Vena caval flow cannot be assessed on transthoracic echocardiography, but hepatic vein flow provides a useful surrogate. This is assessed from the subcostal view using PW Doppler with the sample volume placed 1 cm within the hepatic vein (Fig. 14.2c). Normal hepatic vein flow is complex, with forward flow occurring predominantly in systole, but also in diastole, with low-velocity flow reversals (Fig. 14.2c).

Right heart blood flow is heavily influenced by respiration such that forward velocities at all sites increase during inspiration.

Tricuspid regurgitation

A trivial amount of tricuspid regurgitation is very common, but moderate/severe regurgitation is always pathological. If you detect tricuspid regurgitation you should aim to assess the severity and identify a potential cause.

Assessing severity

As with any valve lesion, assessment of tricuspid regurgitation severity is based on an integrated interpretation of multiple imaging modalities. This starts with two-dimensional imaging to look for evidence of primary valve pathology and the secondary effects of valve dysfunction on the right chambers of the heart, e.g. right ventricular/atrial dilatation. Next, CFM and spectral Doppler are used to assess the regurgitant jet characteristics, and the effects on inferior vena cava blood flow. Essentially these techniques are analogous to assessment of mitral regurgitation.

Two-dimensional imaging

The appearance of the tricuspid valve is an important clue to the underlying aetiology (Table 14.1), and also gives some idea of the severity of dysfunction.

You should assess whether the leaflets are thin and mobile, and whether there is normal coaptation. The presence of abnormalities such as leaflet restriction, failed coaptation, thickening, vegetation, prolapse, dysplasia and annular dilatation increases the likelihood of significant tricuspid regurgitation.

CFM Doppler

As with any regurgitant jet, CFM Doppler provides a spatial representation of blood velocity, and gives an impression of regurgitation severity. However, great care needs to be exercised, because the appearance of a regurgitant jet is influenced by the ventricular pressure driving it. In the presence of pulmonary hypertension, right ventricular systolic pressure (RVSP) is high, and tricuspid regurgitation may

Table 14.1 Causes of tricuspid regurgitation

Aetiology	Valve appearance
Primary	
Carcinoid	Leaflet thickening + restriction
Ebstein's anomaly	Dysplastic leaflet(s) with apical displacement
Endocarditis	Vegetation
Endomyocardial fibrosis	Leaflet and endocardial thickening + restriction
Prolapse	Leaflet thickening, segmental prolapse, often associated mitral valve prolapse
Pacing wires	Chronic pacing lead
Rheumatic	Leaflet, chordal and commissural thickening, calcification and restriction
Ventricular septal defect	Perimembranous ventricular septal defect + septal leaflet aneurysm closing defect
Secondary	
Functional	Structurally normal valve + right ventricular dilatation due to other cause

appear more dramatic than at lower pressures. In addition, the well-recognised effects of gain settings and aliasing velocity make the appearance even more variable. Therefore simple CFM Doppler measures such as jet length and area are not recommended.

Analysis of the proximal isovelocity surface area (PISA) radius and vena contracta width provides more robust measures of tricuspid regurgitation severity (Fig. 14.3). The methods used are identical to those applied to other valves. A useful rule of thumb is that severe tricuspid regurgitation has a PISA radius of >9 mm at an aliasing velocity of 40 cm/s, and a vena contracta width of ≥7 mm. This is analogous to using PISA lite for assessing mitral regurgitation.

Spectral Doppler

CW Doppler aligned with the turbulent high-velocity flow at the vena contracta of the regurgitant jet provides a semiquantitative estimate of severity. The intensity of the spectrum of the regurgitant flow is compared to forward flow. In mild tricuspid regurgitation the regurgitant envelope is incomplete and not very dense. As severity worsens the intensity begins to resemble forward flow (Fig. 14.3). In addition, there may be a late systolic blunting of velocity as right atrial pressure equalises with right ventricular pressure: this results in a rather triangular appearance to the profile of the peak velocity.

Figure 14.3

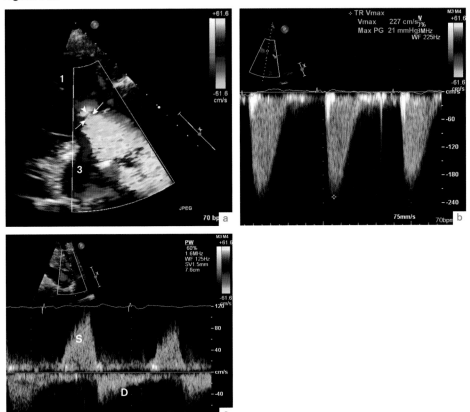

Assessing tricuspid regurgitation severity. (a) Parasternal short axis view. This patient has a dual-chamber pacemaker, with leads in the right ventricle and right atrium. Colour flow mapping Doppler shows a large, broad jet of tricuspid regurgitation. The vena contracta is indicated by the arrows. The proximal isovelocity surface area (PISA) zone is indicated by the abrupt change in colour from blue to yellow (arrowhead). The radius from the PISA to the valve orifice and the peak velocity of the jet (227 cm/s) can be measured, allowing calculation of the effective regurgitant orifice area. **(b)** Continuous wave (CW) Doppler of tricuspid regurgitation. The CW Doppler demonstrates a dense regurgitant jet, consistent with severe regurgitation. The pressure gradient between the right ventricle and atrium is 21 mmHg. **(c)** Hepatic vein pulse wave Doppler: there is systolic flow reversal (S) and diastolic dominant forward flow (D) indicative of severe tricuspid regurgitation.

View **On-line** Images

Secondary features

In cases of primary valvular disease right ventricular dilatation due to volume overload is a sign of significant tricuspid regurgitation.

Significant regurgitation increases right atrial pressure, causing dilatation of the atrium, inferior vena cava and hepatic veins. Blood flow into the right atrium from the major veins usually occurs predominantly in systole: tricuspid regurgitation may cause blunted hepatic vein systolic forward flow, or even systolic flow reversal (Fig. 14.3c).

Figure 14.4

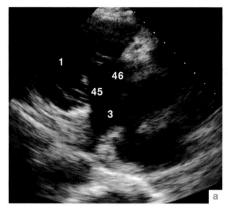
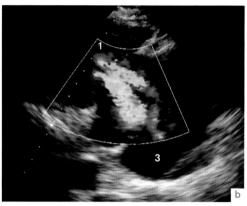

Functional tricuspid regurgitation. (a) There is dilatation of the right ventricle and tricuspid annulus leading to failure of tricuspid valve leaflet coaptation. **(b)** Two jets of tricuspid regurgitation are evident.

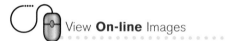
View **On-line** Images

What is the cause?

The commonest situation is functional tricuspid regurgitation secondary to right ventricular dilatation due to any pathological process that causes right heart pressure or volume overload. In this situation you would expect to see a structurally normal tricuspid valve, with a dilated tricuspid annulus and failure of leaflet coaptation (Fig. 14.4).

Primary structural causes are less common, and include Ebstein's anomaly, rheumatic valve disease, carcinoid syndrome and endocarditis. Rheumatic tricuspid degeneration usually occurs in association with left-sided valve lesions (e.g. mitral stenosis), with evidence of commissural fusion, leaflet/chordal thickening, calcification and retraction. Endocarditis of the tricuspid valve occurs particularly in intravenous drug abusers. Perimembranous ventricular septal defects can close by a process that involves the septal leaflet of the tricuspid valve, and may lead to tricuspid regurgitation (Fig. 20.7).

Tricuspid stenosis

Tricuspid stenosis is a rare condition. It can occur as a congenital disorder, but is seen in cases of carcinoid syndrome, rheumatic degeneration or Loeffler's endomyocardial fibrosis. In the past certain appetite-suppressing drugs were a cause. In all of these conditions there is evidence of leaflet thickening and restriction, often with involvement of the subvalvular apparatus (Fig. 14.5). There is often a mixture of stenosis and regurgitation.

The principles of assessment are the same as those of mitral stenosis, except valve orifice planimetry is not performed. PW Doppler interrogation of right ventricular inflow through the tricuspid valve is used to measure:

Figure 14.5

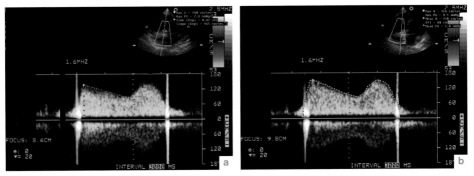

Assessment of tricuspid stenosis. (a) Measurement of the pressure half-time. **(b)** Measurement of mean tricuspid valve gradient.

1. Pressure half-time (Fig. 14.5a): time for the pressure gradient across the tricuspid valve to decrease to half the peak value. Measurement involves measuring the deceleration gradient of early diastolic flow. A pressure half-time >190 ms suggests severe stenosis (valve area <1.0 cm^2).

2. Mean pressure gradient (Fig. 14.5b): the forward-flow Doppler spectrum is traced to obtain mean gradient across the valve: mild, <2 mmHg; moderate, <5 mmHg; severe, >5 mmHg.

In pure tricuspid stenosis the right ventricle is usually normal in structure and function. Secondary features of tricuspid stenosis include right atrial dilatation and evidence of inferior vena caval congestion, with reduced systolic forward flow in the hepatic veins.

Pulmonary stenosis

Pulmonary stenosis can occur as a congenital condition, either in isolation or combination with other congenital cardiac abnormalities. It is particularly associated with Noonan's syndrome, in which there is valvular dysplasia causing abnormal valve thickening. Acquired pulmonary stenosis is rare, occurring secondary to rheumatic heart disease and carcinoid syndrome.

Supravalvular and subvalvular pulmonary stenosis may occur in certain congenital disorders (e.g. tetralogy of Fallot), due to fibromuscular narrowing, and may mimic the Doppler echocardiographic findings of pulmonary valve stenosis.

Assessment of pulmonary stenosis

Valve gradient

Assessment of the transpulmonary valve gradient using the Bernoulli equation is identical to its application to the aortic valve. CW Doppler is aligned with flow through the pulmonary valve, usually from the PSSAX view (Fig. 14.6). Peak velocity is measured: gradient = $4\ V_{max}^2$.

Figure 14.6

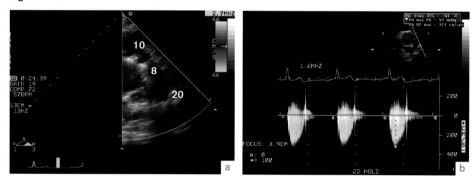

Pulmonary stenosis. This patient underwent a Ross procedure as a child and received a pulmonary homograft. **(a)** The valve is thickened and immobile. **(b)** Continuous wave Doppler shows evidence of pulmonary stenosis and regurgitation. Peak instantaneous gradient is 41 mmHg, indicating mild stenosis.

View **On-line** Images

The ranges for pulmonary stenosis are: mild, <50 mmHg; moderate, ≤80 mmHg; severe, >80 mmHg.

Continuity equation

Pulmonary valve area can be calculated using the continuity equation, as explained in Chapter 12.

$$\text{Pulmonary valve area} = \frac{\text{area}_{RVOT} \times \text{VTI}_{RVOT}}{\text{VTI}_{PV}}$$

where area$_{RVOT}$ is the calculated subpulmonic RVOT area, VTI$_{RVOT}$ is the velocity time integral of flow through the RVOT using PW Doppler, and VTI$_{PV}$ is the velocity time integral of flow through the pulmonary valve using CW Doppler. Peak velocities can be used instead of VTI. Pulmonary valve area can be stratified as follows: mild, 1–2 cm^2; moderate, 0.5–1.0 cm^2; severe, <0.5 cm^2.

Pulmonary regurgitation

Pulmonary valve regurgitation occurs in congenital absence of the pulmonary valve, or congenital valve dysplasia. Causes of acquired pulmonary regurgitation include rheumatic valve disease, carcinoid syndrome, infective endocarditis, pulmonary annulus dilatation secondary to pulmonary hypertension and Marfan's syndrome.

Assessment of pulmonary regurgitation

Pulmonary regurgitation can be detected using CFM Doppler in the PSSAX view (Fig. 14.7a). This can then be used to align spectral Doppler with the regurgitant

Figure 14.7

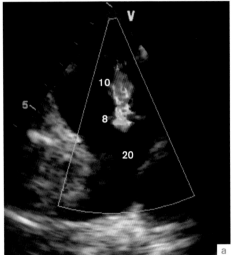

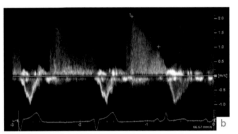

Pulmonary regurgitation. (a) Parasternal short axis view. Colour flow mapping Doppler. There is a narrow central pulmonary regurgitant jet. **(b)** Continuous wave Doppler aligned with regurgitant flow is used to measure the pressure half-time.

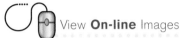 View **On-line** Images

flow (Fig. 14.7b). The assessment of the severity of pulmonary regurgitation is based on similar principles to those applied to aortic regurgitation. As for any valvular lesion, multiple parameters should be taken into account.

Valve appearance

Evidence of severe leaflet abnormality (e.g. failure of coaptation, thickening, destruction) suggests that pulmonary regurgitation is likely to be significant. Also look for evidence of pulmonary annular dilatation.

CFM Doppler

Significant pulmonary regurgitation is suggested by a wide regurgitant jet relative to the RVOT diameter. No specific cut-off values are in widespread use. In addition, a jet length exceeding 20 mm or jet area greater than >1.5 cm² suggests severe regurgitation (Fig. 14.7).

CW Doppler

Equal intensity of the regurgitant signal compared to forward pulmonary flow indicates significant pulmonary regurgitation. The pressure half-time of the regurgitant jet should be measured: mild, >100 ms; moderate and severe, <100 ms.

Quantitative techniques

The regurgitant fraction can be calculated as described in Chapter 11: mild, <40%; moderate, 40–60%; severe, >60%.

Secondary effects

Significant chronic pulmonary regurgitation usually causes right ventricular volume overload, dilatation and hypertrophy.

Diseases of the right heart valves

The tricuspid and pulmonary valves are susceptible to the full range of pathologies that affect other valves, such as endocarditis and rheumatic valve disease. In addition there are some conditions that are specific to each valve and warrant special consideration.

Tricuspid valve prolapse

Prolapse of the tricuspid valve can occur, usually in association with mitral valve prolapse (Chapter 13). It is recognised by similar criteria of valve thickening and leaflet displacement behind the plane of the tricuspid annulus in the A4C view (Fig. 14.8).

Carcinoid syndrome

Carcinoid heart disease is characterised by extensive valvular fibrosis particularly affecting the tricuspid and pulmonary valves. Leaflets become thickened and completely immobile, leading to severe valvular regurgitation, and sometimes stenosis

Figure 14.8

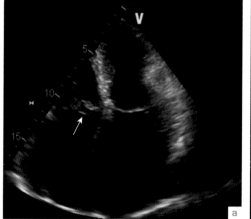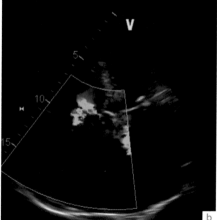

Tricuspid valve prolapse. (a and **b)** Apical four-chamber view. There is prolapse of the posterior leaflet of the tricuspid valve causing mild tricuspid regurgitation.

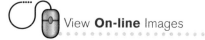 View **On-line** Images

Figure 14.9

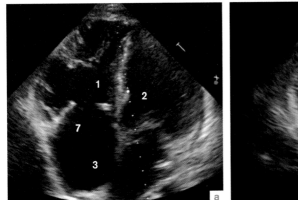
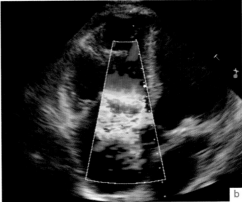

Carcinoid heart disease. (a and **b)** Apical four-chamber view. The tricuspid valve leaflets are thickened and held rigidly open in mid-systole, causing both tricuspid stenosis and regurgitation. There is also severe right ventricular dilatation.

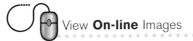 View **On-line** Images

(Fig. 14.9). It is caused by excessive levels of serotonin secreted by carcinoid tumours arising within the gut. Left-sided valve disease may occur with pulmonary carcinoid tumours. Certain drugs, previously used as appetite suppressants, have been shown to cause similar valvular problems.

Ebstein's anomaly

This is a congenital abnormality of the tricuspid valve, in which there is displacement of the septal leaflet of the tricuspid valve towards the apex of the heart (more than 8 mm difference compared to the mitral valve), with 'atrialisation' of a portion of ventricle. The other leaflets may or may not be displaced. The leaflets are often structurally abnormal (dysplastic), causing tricuspid regurgitation, which may eventually cause right ventricular and atrial dilatation (Fig. 14.10).

Although this is a congenital condition, some cases present in adulthood with evidence of right heart failure. It is also associated with Wolff–Parkinson–White syndrome, with a right-sided accessory atrioventricular conduction pathway.

Assessment of right heart pressures

Important haemodynamic information about right heart function is available from routine Doppler examination of the tricuspid and pulmonary valves. It is possible to estimate pulmonary artery, right ventricular and right atrial pressure from a standard echo examination with relative ease. When there is severe right heart valve dysfunction the assumptions on which these estimates are based may not be valid and caution should be exercised.

Figure 14.10

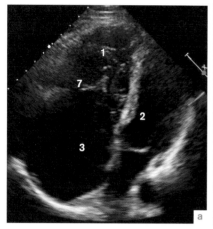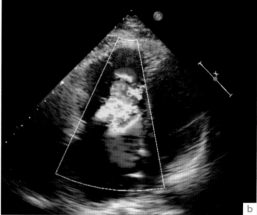

Ebstein's anomaly. (**a** and **b**) Apical four-chamber views. The tricuspid valve is displaced apically, and is severely abnormal in appearance. There is severe tricuspid regurgitation.

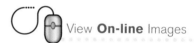 View **On-line** Images

Figure 14.11

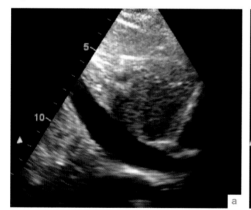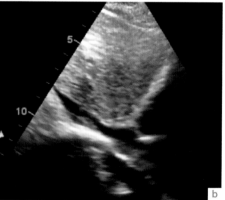

Estimating right atrial pressure. Subcostal views. The diameter and collapsibility of the inferior vena cava are measured during normal respiration (**a**) and after sniffing (**b**). In this case right atrial pressure is 5–10 mmHg.

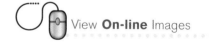 View **On-line** Images

Right atrial pressure

Right atrial pressure is an important haemodynamic parameter as it reflects the degree of venous filling, right ventricular function and the significance of right heart valve disease. It can be assessed quite simply by measuring the dimensions and collapsibility of the inferior vena cava in the subcostal view (Fig. 14.11). If

Table 14.2 Assessment of right atrial pressure from inferior vena cava (IVC) physiology

IVC diameter (cm)	Collapse	Mean right atrial pressure (mmHg)
<1.5	Collapse	0–5
1.5–2.5	>50%	5–10
1.5–2.5	<50%	10–15
>2.5	<50%	15–20
>2.5	No collapse	>20

right atrial pressure is normal, the intrahepatic inferior vena caval diameter will be normal (<2.5 cm), and will demonstrate collapse during inspiration. Sharp inspiration, such as sniffing, is the best test for collapsibility (Fig. 14.11). Inferior vena caval distension and reduced collapse are indicators of raised right atrial pressure, as indicated in Table 14.2.

Right ventricular systolic pressure

RVSP can only be estimated if there is detectable tricuspid regurgitation, as the velocity of this jet reflects the pressure driving it, according to the Bernoulli equation (Fig. 14.12). The peak velocity of the tricuspid regurgitant jet reflects the gradient between the right ventricle and the right atrium, rather than the peak right ventricular pressure itself. Hence:

RVSP = tricuspid regurgitation jet gradient + right atrial pressure

Although tricuspid regurgitation is almost universally present, it can be difficult to record the peak velocity on trivial jets accurately.

Pulmonary artery systolic pressure

Pulmonary artery systolic pressure (PASP) can be estimated by two techniques. The first method relies on the fact that PASP and right ventricular pressure equalise in systole. Assuming there is no obstruction between the right ventricle and pulmonary artery (e.g. pulmonary valve stenosis):

PASP = RVSP = tricuspid regurgitation jet gradient + right atrial pressure

Approximate ranges for pulmonary artery pressure are given in Table 14.3. In practice there are no agreed standards for the exact cut-offs between categories, and it is well recognised that elderly people often have raised pulmonary artery pressure, without other evidence of pathology.

The second method is measurement of pulmonary acceleration time, which is particularly useful in patients who do not have detectable tricuspid regurgitation. This is measured from the onset of pulmonary flow to the peak systolic velocity

Figure 14.12

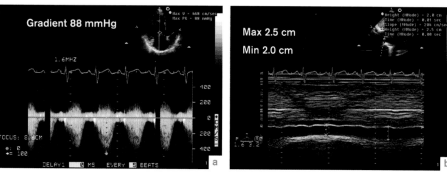

Measuring pulmonary artery systolic pressure. (a) Continuous wave Doppler of tricuspid regurgitant jet. **(b)** M-mode of inferior vena cava (IVC). The systolic pulmonary artery pressure is the sum of the pressure gradient across the tricuspid valve (88 mmHg) and the right atrial pressure (10–15 mmHg).

Table 14.3 Categorisation of pulmonary artery systolic pressure

Category	Pressure (mmHg)
Normal	<35
Mild	<45
Moderate	<60
Severe	≥60

(Fig. 14.2b): >140 ms indicates normal pulmonary artery pressure whilst <90 ms correlates with a PASP in excess of 70 mmHg.

Pulmonary artery diastolic pressure

It is only possible to assess pulmonary artery diastolic pressure if there is pulmonary valve regurgitation. The velocity of regurgitant blood flow between the pulmonary artery and right ventricle depends on the pressure difference between them during diastole. This gradient can be calculated by the Bernoulli equation, using the end diastolic pulmonary regurgitant velocity. To calculate the actual value of pulmonary artery diastolic pressure the right ventricular end diastolic pressure (RVEDP) must be taken into account as well, as this influences the gradient. It cannot be measured directly by echo, but RVEDP must be equal to right atrial pressure, assuming no tricuspid stenosis. Hence:

Pulmonary artery end diastolic pressure $= 4V^2 +$ right atrial pressure

where V is the end diastolic velocity of pulmonary regurgitation jet (Fig. 14.13).

Figure 14.13

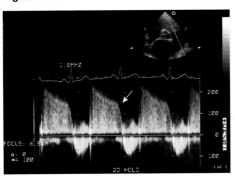

Measuring pulmonary artery diastolic pressure. Continuous wave Doppler is aligned with pulmonary regurgitant flow. The end diastolic velocity (arrow) can be used to calculate diastolic pulmonary artery pressure.

Reporting box

Reporting on tricuspid regurgitation

Summary

- Severity
- Underlying diagnosis/mechanism

Qualitative data

- Leaflet structure, e.g. normal, prolapse, thickening, calcification, vegetations, perforation
- Leaflet mobility, e.g. flail leaflet, restriction
- Structure of subvalvular apparatus and annulus, e.g. thickening, rupture
- Jet characteristics: number, central, eccentric, wall impinging, extent
- Continuous wave Doppler characteristics

Quantitative data

- Vena contracta width
- Proximal isovelocity surface area (PISA) radius (aliasing velocity at 40 cm/s)
- Effective regurgitant orifice area (EROA)
- Regurgitant fraction/volume

Other

- Pulmonary artery pressure
- Right ventricular dimensions and function
- Right atrial dimension
- Inferior vena cava diameter and collapsibility
- Hepatic vein flow pattern

Reporting box

Reporting on tricuspid stenosis

Summary

- Severity
- Underlying diagnosis

Qualitative data

- Leaflet structure, e.g. thickening, calcification
- Leaflet function, e.g. restricted mobility
- Subvalvular structure and function

Quantitative data

- Pressure half-time
- Mean gradient

Other

- Associated valvular lesions, e.g. tricuspid regurgitation
- Right ventricular dimensions
- Right atrial dimensions
- Inferior vena cava diameter
- Hepatic vein flow pattern

Reporting box

Reporting on pulmonary regurgitation

Summary

- Severity
- Underlying diagnosis/mechanism

Qualitative data

- Pulmonary valve structure, e.g. normal, thickening, calcification, vegetations, perforation, failed coaptation, annular dilatation
- Pulmonary valve function
- Jet characteristics: number, central, eccentric, wall impinging, posterior extent
- Continuous wave Doppler characteristics

Quantitative data

- Jet length/area
- Jet width/right ventricular outflow tract width
- Pressure half-time
- Regurgitant fraction/volume

Other

- Pulmonary artery pressure
- Pulmonary artery dimension
- Dimensions of right atrium, ventricle, inferior vena cava, pulmonary artery
- Right ventricular function
- Hepatic vein flow pattern
- Associated valvular lesions

Reporting box

Reporting on pulmonary stenosis

Summary

- Severity
- Underlying diagnosis

Qualitative data

- Valve structure
- Calcification: severity and distribution
- Cusp opening: degree of restriction

Quantitative data

- Peak velocity
- Peak gradient
- Mean gradient
- Estimated valve area

Other

- Right ventricular dimensions
- Right ventricular hypertrophy
- Pulmonary artery dimension
- Associated valvular lesions
- Evidence of sub-/supravalvular stenosis

Infective endocarditis

Infective endocarditis (IE) is usually a bacterial infection of the valves or endocardium of the heart. It is a serious condition that requires early recognition, prompt and appropriate antibiotic therapy, and sometimes valve replacement. In the majority of cases a pre-existing structural abnormality is present that predisposes to infection. Prosthetic material in or near the heart (e.g. central line, pacing wire, artificial heart valve) may also be prone to infection and can have similar consequences.

Diagnosis

The hallmark of IE is a vegetation, which is an infected mass of fibrin attached to a valve or other part of the endocardium. Typically this is a pedunculated mass with independent mobility to the valve (Fig. 15.1). The oscillating movement of a vegetation may be better appreciated by slowly scrolling through the movie: you should carefully review the web images of this chapter to observe this.

In the appropriate clinical context a vegetation provides major evidence for endocarditis, but the converse is not true: the absence of a demonstrable vegetation does not exclude a diagnosis of IE. Transthoracic echocardiography (TTE) cannot reliably detect vegetations <2 mm in diameter, and typical vegetations are not always present. Sometimes the infection forms a sessile mass or generalised valvular thickening that leads to valve dysfunction or destruction (Fig. 15.1c and d). Vegetations do not always regress despite successful treatment, so the presence of a vegetation may simply represent a previous episode of IE.

Hence the diagnosis of IE is not based solely on the identification of a vegetation, but on the overall clinical picture, including the isolation of typical microorganisms from blood cultures. If suspicion is high, and a transthoracic study is

Figure 15.1

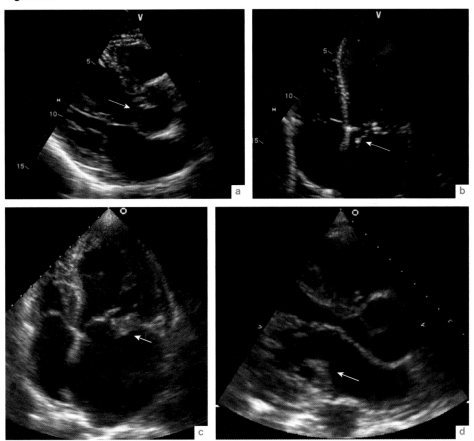

Examples of vegetations. (a) A small pedunculated vegetation is attached to the aortic valve (arrow). **(b)** Large pedunculated vegetation on the anterior mitral valve leaflet. **(c)** Sessile vegetation on the anterior mitral valve leaflet (arrow). **(d)** Posterior mitral valve leaflet thickening in a case of *Staphylococcus aureus* endocarditis. The leaflet is markedly abnormal, and after a few days a large vegetation had developed.

View **On-line** Images

inconclusive, transoesophageal echocardiography (TOE) should be undertaken. This is particularly the case for patients with prosthetic valves, since these can rarely be adequately visualised by TTE.

The commonest sites of infection are the aortic and mitral valves. Multivalvular involvement is uncommon, but a thorough examination of all valves is required once a diagnosis of IE is made. In cases of congenital heart disease shunts and artificial conduits are possible sites of infection. In some centres all patients with IE undergo TOE early in the course of treatment to define the burden of disease and exclude unsuspected complications.

It is important to remember that conditions other than IE can cause valvular masses (Table 15.1). The differential diagnosis is quite broad, and generally it is

Table 15.1 Differential diagnosis of a valvular mass

Differential diagnosis	Features
Active infective endocarditis	Evidence of valve destruction, positive blood cultures
Treated infective endocarditis	Previous history of IE. Calcified vegetation
Marantic endocarditis	Evidence of malignancy/immune disease
Libman–Sacks endocarditis	Evidence of SLE. Often sessile
Rheumatic valvulitis	Thickened valve tips. Clinical features of acute rheumatic fever
Chordal rupture	Underlying MVP
Fibroelastoma	Mostly AV or MV. Frond-like appearance with stalk (Fig. 18.7). Valve otherwise normal. High embolic potential
Lambl's excrescence	Degenerative lesion at coaptation point of AV or MV. <2 mm in size (not usually seen with TTE). No valve dysfunction
Atrial myxoma	Rarely valvular. Usually attached to interatrial septum (Fig. 18.1)
Thrombus	Usually mural (Fig. 18.6)

IE, infective endocarditis; SLE, systemic lupus erythematosus; MVP, mitral valve prolapse; AV, aortic valve; MV, mitral valve; TTE, transthoracic echocardiography.

not possible to distinguish lesions based on appearances alone. Usually other clinical information will point towards a particular cause.

Complications

Abscess formation

Abscess formation occurs when valvular infection spreads to the surrounding paravalvular structures and myocardium, forming a discrete collection of pus. It usually appears as an area of perivalvular thickening with echodense areas or an echolucent cavity. It is important to recognize, as antibiotic therapy is likely to fail and valve replacement is usually required. The commonest sites are the aortic root (Fig. 15.2) and the mitral annulus. It may lead to other complications, such as complete heart block and fistula formation.

Valve destruction

IE may lead to valvular dysfunction either by leaflet destruction causing perforation/flail leaflet (Fig. 15.3) or chordal rupture. This will invariably cause regurgitation, which may be catastrophic.

Figure 15.2

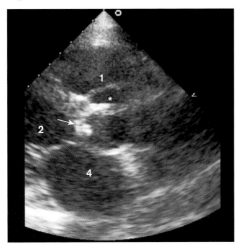

Aortic root abscess. Parasternal long axis view. The non-coronary cusp of the aortic valve is abnormally thickened (arrow), as is the surrounding tissue of the aortic root. An echolucent area, representing an abscess (*), is present between the aortic root and the right ventricle.

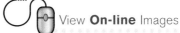

View **On-line** Images

Figure 15.3

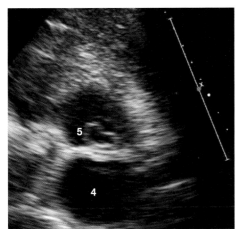

Perforation of the aortic valve. Magnified parasternal short axis view.

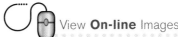

View **On-line** Images

Seeding

Secondary lesions are sometimes spread by regurgitant jets to other valves or non-valvular endocardium (Fig. 15.4).

Embolic complications

Large vegetations (>10 mm) may be more prone to embolisation (Fig. 15.5). Therefore the dimensions of a vegetation should be measured in several views.

Prosthetic valve dehiscence

Infection of a prosthetic valve can lead to destruction of the sutures and tissues attaching the valve casing to the valvular annulus. This may be recognised as a

Figure 15.4

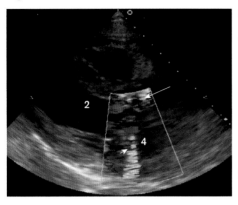

Secondary endocarditis lesion. Parasternal long axis view. Aortic valve endocarditis with severe aortic regurgitation (arrow). The regurgitant jet impinges on the anterior mitral valve leaflet which has perforated, leading to a secondary jet of mitral regurgitation (arrowhead).

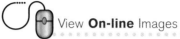

View **On-line** Images

Figure 15.5

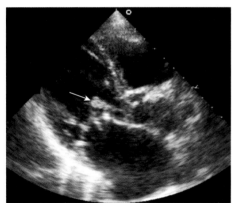

Large vegetation. A 2-cm-long vegetation on the aortic valve.

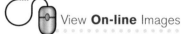

View **On-line** Images

paraprosthetic leak, rocking of the valve or gross movement of the valve independently of the surrounding tissue (dehiscence). Although this situation can be chronic and may arise in the absence of infection, the detection of new valve dehiscence is highly suggestive of IE. Other implanted material, such as annuloplasty rings and pacemaker wires, can also become infected (Fig. 15.6).

Detection of a predisposing condition

It is unusual for completely normal heart valves to become infected, except with particularly virulent organisms such as *Staphylococcus aureus*. The risk of endocarditis depends on the underlying structural abnormality and is highest for patients with previous episodes of endocarditis, prosthetic valves and uncorrected cyanotic congenital heart disease. Guidelines vary around the world regarding the appropriateness of antibiotic prophylaxis for bacteraemia-prone procedures (e.g. dental treatment).

Figure 15.6

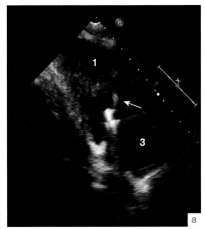

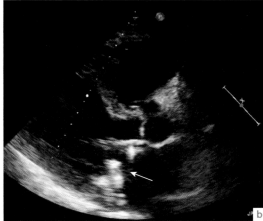

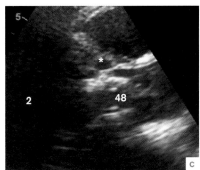

Endocarditis affecting intracardiac prosthetic material. (a) Infected pacing wire in the right ventricle (arrow). **(b)** Infected mitral annular ring following mitral valve repair. Note the evidence of ring dehiscence. **(c)** Vegetation on a bioprosthetic aortic valve replacement (arrow), with evidence of aortic root abscess (*).

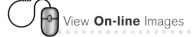 View **On-line** Images

Reporting box

Reporting on possible endocarditis

Summary

- Likely diagnosis
- Valve(s) affected
- Complications
- Need for further investigation, e.g. transoesophageal echocardiography (TOE)

Qualitative data

- Valve affected
- Leaflet/cusp affected
- Leaflet integrity: intact, regurgitation, perforation, flail, dehiscence
- Abscess
- Non-valvular involvement

Quantitative data

- Vegetation dimensions

Other

- Assessment of regurgitation severity

Prosthetic valves

Types of prosthetic valve

The bewildering array of prosthetic valves can be classified into two main categories: mechanical and bioprosthetic (Fig. 16.1). For the purposes of the echocardiographer it is only necessary to have a working knowledge of different valve types and general principles of assessing prosthesis function.

Mechanical valves

Mechanical prostheses are constructed from metal alloys, but sometimes have non-metal components. Valve design has evolved over time, but valves all share a basic construction, with a fabric sewing ring that allows the surgeon to attach the valve to tissue, the valve housing and the occluder mechanism, which allows unidirectional blood flow. The main differences lie in the occluder mechanism. The earliest design in the 1960s was the ball and cage (e.g. Starr–Edwards valve), and a few patients still have these implants. This design was superseded by the single tilting disc (e.g. Björk–Shiley), and then the bileaflet tilting disc (Figs 16.1–16.3). The bileaflet design is most commonly used at present, as this has the most favourable haemodynamic characteristics.

Bioprosthetic valves

Bioprosthetic valves may be obtained from a variety of sources. These include intact valves removed from human cadavers (allograft) and pigs (xenograft). Valves can also be constructed from pericardial tissue (e.g. bovine) mounted in a framework according to various designs (e.g. Carpentier–Edwards, Ionescu, Wessex). In general, bioprosthetic valve types are not echocardiographically distinguishable, except

Figure 16.1

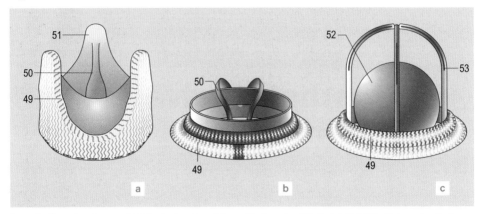

Prosthetic valve types. (a) Stented pericardial prosthetic valve (St Jude). **(b)** Bileaflet mechanical valve (Sorin). **(c)** Starr–Edwards prosthetic valve.

Figure 16.2

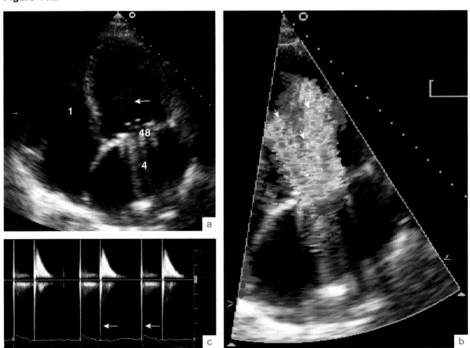

Mitral bileaflet mechanical prosthesis. Apical four-chamber view. **(a)** The mitral bileaflet prosthesis casts an extensive shadow of reverberation artefact into the left atrium, completely obscuring other structures. In addition, a group of microbubbles is seen in the left ventricle (arrow). **(b)** Due to the design of this prosthesis there are three jets of forward flow (arrows). **(c)** Continuous wave Doppler: blood flow across the valve prosthesis is assessed in the same manner as a native valve, e.g. pressure half-time, mean gradient. Note the artefacts generated by opening and closing (arrows).

View **On-line** Images

Figure 16.3

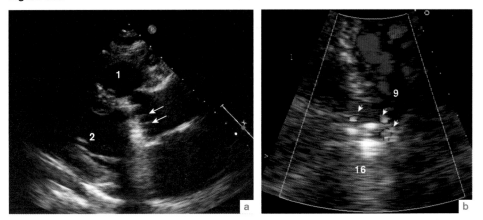

Aortic bileaflet mechanical prosthesis. (a) Parasternal long axis view. **(b)** Apical five-chamber view colour flow mapping Doppler (magnified). Two mechanical leaflets are clearly seen (arrows). During diastole three distinct washout jets are apparent (arrows). These are entirely normal for this type of valve.

View **On-line** Images

that most have an artificial housing/sewing ring (stented bioprosthesis) (see Fig. 16.8, below), which is echoreflective, whilst stentless valves do not.

Normal function

Appearance

Assessment of prosthesis function begins with the valve appearance. Mechanical valves and stented bioprostheses are highly echoreflective, so the valve construction and surrounding structures are often totally obscured. Indeed, acoustic shadowing and reverberations can create artefacts and make valve assessment difficult (Fig. 16.2). Different mechanical valve designs have characteristic appearances, but the level of artefact is such that it is not always possible to identify the type with complete certainty.

Surgical repair of native valves, particularly mitral valve prolapse, is quite common, and often involves implantation of a plastic ring to support the mitral annulus (Fig. 16.4).

You should start by identifying the type of prosthesis, its location and whether it is well seated or not. Next, look for moving parts – leaflets, discs or balls – and decide if there is any abnormal, delayed or restricted movement. Finally, look for evidence of abnormal structures attached to the valve, such as thrombus, pannus or vegetations. Small filamentous lesions can sometimes form on prosthetic valves, and are considered normal. Surgical stitches protruding from the sewing ring may occasionally be seen, but can be difficult to differentiate from thrombus and vegetations. Finally small bubbles can sometimes be seen, which are probably microcavitations caused by turbulence around metallic components of the valve (Fig. 16.2). These are entirely normal.

Figure 16.4

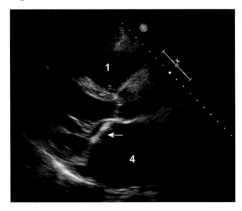

Mitral annular ring. Parasternal long axis view. This patient has undergone mitral valve repair, including implantation of a plastic ring (arrow) to prevent annular dilatation.

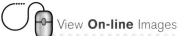 View **On-line** Images

Function

Prosthetic valve function should be assessed in the same manner as a native valve using the full range of Doppler modalities. Unfortunately, prosthetic valves do not completely replicate normal valve function, and there is usually some obstruction to flow. This should be assessed with continuous wave Doppler using the same principles as applied to native valve assessment. Normal ranges for each specific valve type and size are available, but a general rule of thumb is that obstruction should be no more than mild using native valve criteria. Moderate obstruction is recognised as normal for older valve designs such as the Starr–Edwards valve. Because prosthetic valve orifices can be complex, with multiple distinct jets (Fig. 16.2), an accurate estimate of the valvular gradient/valve area can be difficult. There is usually a systematic overestimate of bileaflet prosthesis transvalvular gradient because the central orifice formed between the two tilting discs is usually smaller than the lateral orifices between the discs and the valve housing.

A trace of valvular regurgitation is also common, particularly with bileaflet valves, which are designed to have small regurgitant 'washout' jets to reduce the risk of valve thrombosis (Fig. 16.3b).

Abnormal prosthetic valve function

Paravalvular regurgitation

Regurgitation of blood around the valve housing, rather than through the valve, is always abnormal (Fig. 16.5). It indicates detachment of the sewing ring from the surrounding tissue, which may be due to a variety of factors, such as infection, friable paravalvular tissue or poor suturing. The significance depends on the severity of regurgitation, stability of the valve position and underlying cause. Mild or moderate paravalvular regurgitation may be well tolerated if it does not worsen and there is no infection. However, progressive deterioration may necessitate re-do surgery.

Figure 16.5

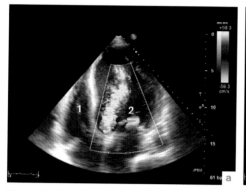
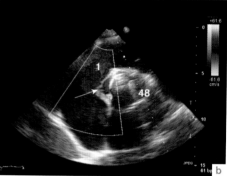

Paravalvular regurgitation. (a) Apical five-chamber colour flow mapping (CFM) Doppler.
(b) Parasternal short axis (PSSAX) CFM Doppler. A Starr–Edwards valve is in the aortic position.
(a) CFM Doppler suggests severe prosthetic
valve regurgitation. **(b)** The PSSAX view
demonstrates that the regurgitant jet
originates from outside the prosthesis (arrow).   View **On-line** Images

Figure 16.6

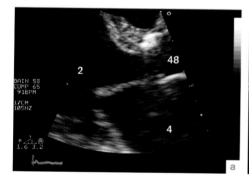
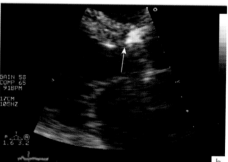

Prosthetic valve dehiscence. Parasternal long axis view (magnified). Separation between the aortic
prosthesis and paravalvular tissue can be seen at
different phases of the cardiac cycle (arrow). This
rocking motion is best appreciated from the
accompanying movie file.   View **On-line** Images

Reverberation artefacts can hinder accurate localisation and characterisation of regurgitant jets on both transthoracic echocardiography (TTE) and transoesophageal echocardiography (TOE).

Dehiscence

Suture dehiscence is a serious situation that invariably requires prosthesis replacement. It is recognised by instability or rocking of the prosthesis (Fig. 16.6). It may be associated with paravalvular regurgitation, and is often due to paravalvular infection or progressive haemodynamic stress on weakened sutures.

Pannus

Pannus is a term used to describe fibrous growth around and sometimes within a prosthetic valve. It is a complication that develops over years, and can lead to leaflet obstruction, causing either regurgitation or stenosis.

Thrombus

All mechanical valve prostheses are prone to thrombosis, though it is more common for the older designs and tricuspid/mitral prostheses as blood flow velocities are relatively low. Consequences include acute valve obstruction, valvular stenosis or regurgitation, and emboli. Thrombus may be directly evident on a leaflet, or inferred from reduced leaflet mobility.

Endocarditis

A high level of suspicion for prosthetic valve endocarditis should be maintained. It can be manifest by the presence of vegetations (Fig. 15.6), which may cause valvular dysfunction (regurgitation, or stenosis), paravalvular abscess, paravalvular regurgitation or dehiscence. It is notoriously difficult to visualise prosthetic valves adequately using TTE, so TOE is mandatory in cases of suspected prosthetic valve endocarditis.

Percutaneous valve treatments

A recent advance has been the development of percutaneous techniques to treat valvular heart disease in patients who are otherwise unsuitable for a conventional valve replacement operation. The increasing use of these techniques means that patients with these devices will inevitably require echocardiographic follow-up.

Specially designed bioprostheses can be used to treat aortic stenosis (transaortic valve implantation) (Fig. 16.7). A percutaneous pulmonary valve implant is also

Figure 16.7

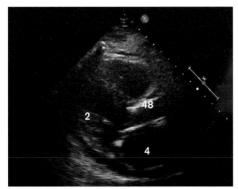

Transaortic valve implant. Parasternal long axis view. This patient has undergone percutaneous implantation of a bioprosthetic aortic valve. The metal housing to the valve is clearly seen protruding into the left ventricular outflow tract.

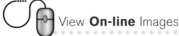

View **On-line** Images

Figure 16.8

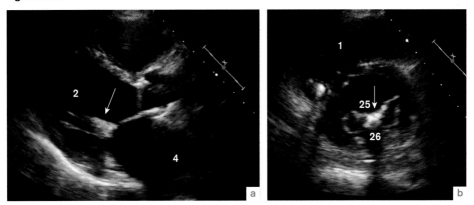

MitraClip device. (a) Parasternal long axis view. **(b)** Parasternal short axis (PSSAX) view. A clip (arrow) has been attached to the mitral valve leaflet tips to improve central coaptation. This effectively results in two valve orifices on the PSSAX view. Note that the patient also has a stented bioprosthetic aortic valve.

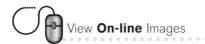 View **On-line** Images

available for the treatment of pulmonary regurgitation in patients who have had previous surgical correction of congenital heart disease.

Mitral regurgitation can sometimes be treated percutaneously with a MitraClip device that tethers the leaflet tips together, improving coaptation (Fig. 16.8).

Reporting box

Reporting on prosthetic valves

Summary

- Type of valve prosthesis
- Normal or abnormal function
- Severity of dysfunction
- Recommendation for further investigation

Qualitative data

- Position of valve
- Stability, seating of valve
- Presence of regurgitation: valvular, paravalvular, central, eccentric, washout
- Presence of obstruction or abnormal leaflet mobility
- Abnormal masses, e.g. vegetation, thrombus, pannus, stitch

Quantitative data

- Peak velocity/mean gradient across valve
- Parameters of regurgitation severity

Pericardial disease

Introduction

The pericardium is a fibroelastic protective covering that surrounds the heart. It has a tough fibrous outer layer and two thin inner layers that form a lubricating sac. Echocardiography is invaluable for detecting pericardial disease and the physiological effects of this on cardiac function.

Echocardiographic appearance

The pericardium is easily identified as an echo-bright structure surrounding the heart in most views. Normally there is minimal separation of this from the adjacent myocardium (Fig. 17.1). Sometimes epicardial fat is present, separating the myocardium and pericardium. This has a granular or speckled appearance (Fig. 17.2) and is more common in the elderly, particularly those with obesity and diabetes.

Pericarditis, pericardial effusion and tamponade

A wide variety of pathologies can cause pericarditis and this often leads to the development of a pericardial effusion (Table 17.1). The majority of pericardial effusions in developed countries are caused by benign self-limiting viral infections, but not all cases develop a detectable pericardial effusion, so the lack of an effusion does not exclude the diagnosis of pericarditis if other clinical features are consistent with this.

A pericardial effusion is an abnormal accumulation of fluid in the pericardial sac (Fig. 17.3). It appears as a dark echo-free space between the pericardium and myocardium, and can usually be seen most easily on the subcostal view. It is not

Figure 17.1

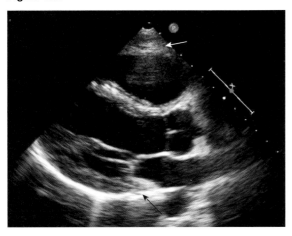

Normal pericardium. Parasternal long axis view. Normal pericardium appears echo-bright (arrows).

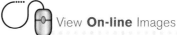
View **On-line** Images

Figure 17.2

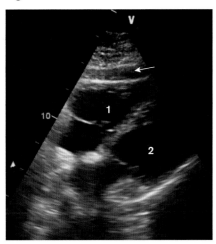

Pericardial fat. Subcostal view. Typical speckled appearance of pericardial fat (arrow).

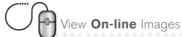
View **On-line** Images

Figure 17.3

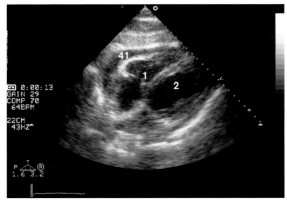

Pericardial effusion. Subcostal view. There is a small pericardial effusion around the right ventricular free wall.

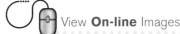
View **On-line** Images

Table 17.1 Causes of pericardial effusion

	Common	Rare
Infective	Viral	Tuberculosis
		Bacterial
		Fungal
Malignant	Lung, breast, lymphoma	
Inflammatory	Dressler's syndrome	Systemic lupus erythematosus
	Post cardiac surgery	Rheumatoid arthritis, Scleroderma
		Sarcoidosis
Other	Heart failure	Uraemia
		Aortic dissection
		Trauma
		Hypothyroidism

Figure 17.4

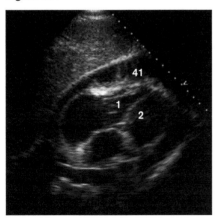

Pericardial fibrin strands. Subcostal view. Dense fibrin strands are present in the pericardial effusion.

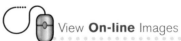
View **On-line** Images

usually possible to identify the cause of a pericardial effusion from the echo appearances. The presence of fibrin strands suggests an inflammatory/infective cause but is not diagnostic (Fig. 17.4).

Differential diagnosis

The appearances of a pericardial effusion must be distinguished from a left-sided pleural effusion and epicardial fat. In general pericardial effusions surround the

Figure 17.5

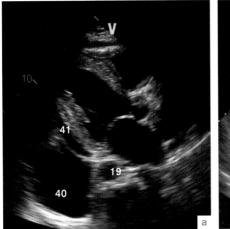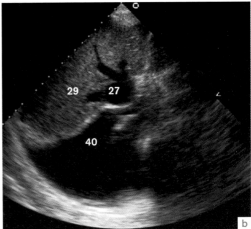

Pleural effusions. (a) Parasternal long axis view. There is a small pericardial effusion and a large pleural effusion: note the relative positions in relation to the descending aorta. **(b)** Subcostal view. Right-sided pleural effusion.

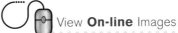 View **On-line** Images

atria and lead to separation of the heart and descending aorta, whereas pleural effusions do not (Fig. 17.5a). However, the distinction may not always be so straightforward, and of course the two may coexist. Right-sided pleural effusions are easily identified from the subcostal view (Fig. 17.5b), appearing as an echo-free space adjacent to the liver.

Assessment of pericardial effusions

Pericardial effusions are a relatively common finding, and an evaluation of the physiological significance of an effusion must be made. This involves assessment of pericardial fluid depth/volume, localisation and signs of cardiac tamponade.

Depth

The maximal depth of a circumferential effusion should be measured in diastole. It is a rough guide to the volume of fluid: <1 cm, small (<100 ml); <2 cm, moderate (<500 ml); >2 cm, large (>500 ml).

Localisation

In general most pericardial effusions affect the whole pericardial space (Fig. 17.6), but adhesions within the pericardial space may restrict the effusion to one particular area (Fig. 17.7). This is more commonly seen after cardiac surgery. In this context a wide range of echocardiographic views should be obtained to identify a loculated effusion.

Figure 17.6

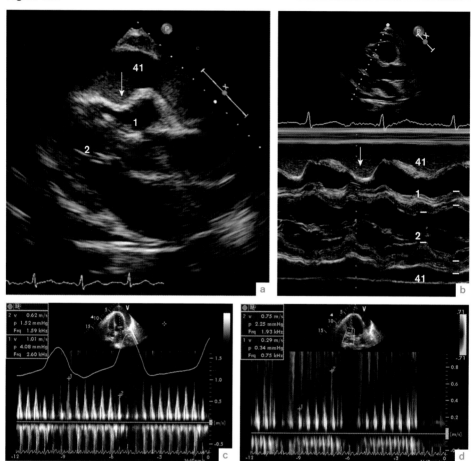

Cardiac tamponade. (a) Parasternal long axis (PSLAX) view. There is a large pericardial effusion, which can be seen to cause collapse of the right ventricle (arrow) during diastole. **(b)** PSLAX M-mode confirms right ventricular collapse (arrow). **(c)** Mitral inflow continuous wave (CW) Doppler: there is a marked increase in peak early inflow velocity with expiration. Peak velocity declines with inspiration. **(d)** Tricuspid inflow CW Doppler: the opposite respiratory effects are observed.

View **On-line** Images

Tamponade

Cardiac tamponade occurs when the heart is compressed by pericardial fluid. This occurs when the intrapericardial pressure exceeds the diastolic pressure of the cardiac chambers, and can occur with an effusion of any size. It is an emergency because it can lead to cardiac arrest if left untreated.

In the commonest situation a large pericardial effusion develops slowly and compensatory distension of the fibrous pericardium accommodates the excess fluid

Figure 17.7

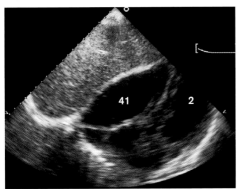

Loculated pericardial effusion. Subcostal view. This patient has a loculated effusion compressing the right ventricle following coronary artery bypass surgery.

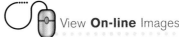 View **On-line** Images

without a major increase in intrapericardial pressure. Eventually pericardial expansion ceases, and further fluid accumulation leads to a significant increase in pressure, causing tamponade. Less commonly a small volume of pericardial fluid may accumulate very rapidly (e.g. ventricular rupture), leading to an acute increase in pericardial pressure and immediate tamponade.

Cardiac tamponade initially compresses the atria as these operate at the lowest pressure. If intrapericardial pressure increases further, right ventricular diastolic compression occurs, and cardiac output is seriously compromised. Superimposed on this is an exaggerated fall in cardiac output during inspiration. In health there is slight variation in cardiac filling with respiration, due to a lowering of intrathoracic pressure during inspiration, which facilitates right heart filling. However, in tamponade the ventricles become 'interdependent' so that right ventricular filling occurs at the expense of left ventricular filling: left ventricular output therefore falls during inspiration, whilst right ventricular output falls during expiration.

Echocardiographic features of cardiac tamponade
Echocardiographic diagnosis of cardiac tamponade requires the demonstration of a pericardial effusion and evidence of excessive respiratory variation in cardiac filling or stroke volume (Fig. 17.6). The earliest sign is diastolic collapse of the atria, though this is not very specific for tamponade. Right ventricular diastolic collapse is more significant, but can be overdiagnosed from a parasternal short axis view of the right ventricular outflow tract.

Significant respiratory variation in cardiac filling is sought by examining the transmitral and tricuspid inflow using pulse wave Doppler. A decrease in trans*mitral* early passive filling (peak E wave) with inspiration of more than 25% is compatible with tamponade. An increase in trans*tricuspid* E wave velocity with inspiration of more than 40% is also significant. Similar variation can be seen in blood flow from the left and right ventricular outflow tracts.

Figure 17.8

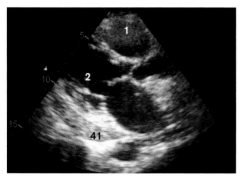

Confirmation of pericardial drain position. Agitated saline injected through a pericardial drain during pericardiocentesis opacifies the pericardial space, confirming that the drain is in the correct location.

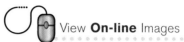

View **On-line** Images

Impaired cardiac filling leads to inferior vena caval dilatation, with predominant systolic forward flow, and expiratory reversal of hepatic vein flow (See constrictive pericarditis section, below).

Echo findings may be modified or atypical in a variety of situations. For example, loculated effusions can be small, and may not cause profound respiratory changes in Doppler parameters. Patients who are on positive-pressure ventilation also lack typical Doppler findings. Conditions which cause raised intracardiac end diastolic pressures (e.g. pre-existing pulmonary/valvular/ myocardial disease) will delay the onset of tamponade, as higher intrapericardial pressure must be reached to cause a haemodynamic effect. Equally, patients with intravascular volume depletion (e.g. dehydration) are prone to tamponade at lower intrapericardial pressure. Finally, pre-existing pericardial thickening may lead to effusive–constrictive physiology (see later).

An additional benefit of echocardiography is that it allows the best approach for percutaneous pericardial drainage (pericardiocentesis) to be determined: either subxiphisternal (subcostal view) or anterior (apical view). A depth of 2 cm or more is usually considered adequate for safe drainage. Echocardiography can also be useful during pericardiocentesis to confirm the drain position: an injection of agitated saline through the drain opacifies the pericardial space (Fig. 17.8).

Constrictive pericarditis

Healthy pericardium is thin (<4 mm) and slightly elastic. Pericardial constriction occurs when the pericardium becomes rigid due to fibrosis and calcification. This can follow pericarditis of virtually any cause, but it is most common after tuberculous pericarditis, radiotherapy or cardiac surgery. Constrictive physiology is sometimes observed as a transient feature during effusive pericarditis.

Constriction usually affects all chambers of the heart, but it is sometimes localised to one region. In some cases the fibrosis and calcification can extend into the epicardial muscle of the heart, causing myocardial dysfunction in addition to pericardial constriction.

Physiology of pericardial constriction

The key to understanding and remembering the echocardiographic features of constrictive pericarditis is to understand the physiology behind it. The fundamental problem is that the heart is encased within the pericardium, preventing full expansion of the cardiac chambers. This means that ventricular filling is prematurely curtailed in early to mid-diastole, and the end diastolic volume is decreased. This reduces cardiac output, causing a pressure increase in all cardiac chambers and their venous connections. The combination of high atrial pressures and limited filling means that blood flow from the atria to the ventricles is of high velocity and short duration.

Pericardial constraint has a number of other effects. Firstly, because the maximal volume of the heart is fixed, the end diastolic pressures in all four cardiac chambers must be equal. It also means that an increase in the volume of one chamber occurs at the expense of the other chambers (interdependence). Secondly, the heart is effectively isolated from respiratory changes in intrathoracic pressure, but the venous and arterial connections of the heart that pass outside the pericardium remain subject to such changes. This results in abnormal patterns of respiratory variation in cardiac filling. For example, during inspiration, left heart filling is reduced, because the reduction in intrathoracic pressure is only transmitted to the pulmonary veins, but not the left atrium. This reduces the pressure gradient for blood flow to the left atrium. The opposite changes occur during right heart filling, i.e. reduced filling in expiration. These effects are reflected in the characteristic features of pericardial constriction (Fig. 17.9).

Two-dimensional and M-mode findings

There is usually evidence of pericardial thickening greater than 4 mm. However, this is an unreliable sign as the appearance is greatly affected by the gain and tissue harmonic settings of the echo machine. Furthermore, pericardial thickening may occur without constrictive physiology, or vice versa.

Abnormal ventricular filling/interdependence causes a characteristic 'septal bounce'. This is due to exaggerated interventricular septal diastolic movement towards the right ventricle. On M-mode the posterior left ventricular wall flattens in mid to late diastole due to interrupted ventricular filling. Raised cardiac pressures cause a variety of abnormalities, including premature mitral valve closure, premature pulmonary valve opening and inferior vena caval dilatation.

Doppler findings

Left ventricular diastolic filling usually has a 'constrictive pattern'. This is characterised by a predominant E wave (>90 cm/s), short deceleration time (<160 ms) and E:A ratio ≥1.5. These findings are similar to a restrictive pattern, but less severe. In the majority of patients myocardial function is normal, reflected by normal tissue Doppler velocities at the lateral mitral annulus (e' peak velocity ≥7 cm/s) with an E/e' ratio of less than 15. A minority of patients have a restrictive filling pattern (Table 17.2).

Figure 17.9

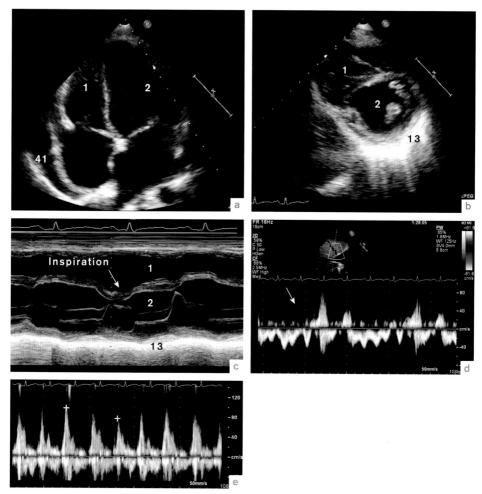

Constrictive pericarditis. (a) Apical four-chamber view. Characteristic interventricular septal bounce. Pericardial fluid is evident around the right atrium. **(b)** Parasternal short axis view. Marked thickening of the posterior pericardium. **(c)** Parasternal long axis M-mode. During inspiration right ventricular filling is augmented at the expense of the left ventricle (arrow). **(d)** Hepatic vein flow: note the marked expiratory diastolic flow reversal (arrow). **(e)** Mitral valve inflow continuous wave Doppler: marked respiratory variation in early diastolic filling.

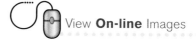 View **On-line** Images

Exaggerated respiratory variation in ventricular filling is invariably seen. This results in a decrease in mitral E wave peak velocity >25% with inspiration. The pattern for right heart filling is an expiratory decrease in tricuspid E wave peak velocity >40%.

Abnormal venous flow into the left atrium is reflected by blunted pulmonary vein systolic flow (systolic:diastolic <1) during inspiration. Hepatic vein flow is also abnormal, with blunted systolic and diastolic forward flow and diastolic end expiratory flow reversal.

Table 17.2 Comparison of echocardiographic findings in pericardial constriction and restrictive cardiomyopathy

Feature	Pericardial constriction	Restrictive cardiomyopathy
Pericardium	Thickened	Normal
Atria	Normal	Enlarged
Left ventricle	Normal	LVH, small LV cavity
LV function	Normal	Diastolic ± systolic dysfunction
Septal motion	Respiratory shift	Normal
Transmitral filling pattern	E:A>1.5 DT <160 ms Abnormal respiratory variation	E:A>1.5 DT <160 ms Normal respiratory variation
Pulmonary vein flow	Systolic dominant	Diastolic dominant
Hepatic vein flow	Expiratory diastolic flow reversal	Inspiratory diastolic flow reversal
Tissue Doppler	Normal velocities	Reduced velocities
	Septal e' ≥7 cm/s	Septal e' <7 cm/s
E/e' ratio	<15	>15

LV, left ventricular; LVH, left ventricular hypertrophy; E:A: ratio of E and A wave peak velocities; DT, E wave deceleration time.

The echocardiographic features of constrictive pericarditis are subtle and may be easily missed. It should therefore be suspected in anyone with a clinical picture of right heart failure (raised jugular venous pressure and peripheral oedema), but normal right ventricular function on echo. However, no single parameter is diagnostic and the whole constellation of abnormalities needs to be taken into account.

Effusive–constrictive pericarditis

This term describes a situation in which there is evidence of both pericardial effusion and pericardial constriction. Usually it is diagnosed after drainage of a pericardial effusion fails to normalise cardiac filling, suggesting that pericardial constriction must be present.

Pericardial constriction versus restrictive cardiomyopathy

The clinical presentations of pericardial constriction and restrictive cardiomyopathy may be similar, because impaired cardiac filling is a feature of both conditions.

It is therefore useful to compare their distinguishing echocardiographic characteristics (Table 17.2). Cardiac muscle function is usually unaffected by pericardial constriction, so tissue Doppler imaging may be the most useful echo parameter. Sometimes it is not possible to make a distinction, and other investigations, such as cardiac catheterisation, cardiac magnetic resonance imaging or computed tomography, are required.

Pericardial tumours

Pericardial tumours are rare and usually spread from other sites, such as lung, breast and oesophagus. The clinical manifestations encompass the whole gamut of pericardial disease, from pericarditis/effusion to tamponade and even pericardial constriction (Fig. 17.10).

Figure 17.10

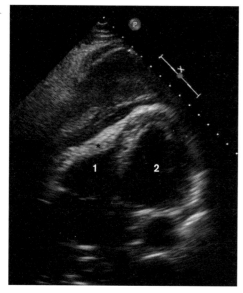

Pericardial tumour. Subcostal view. The pericardium is thickened and echogenic (*) due to an infiltrative lymphoma. There is an obvious 'septal bounce' consistent with constrictive physiology.

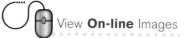

View **On-line** Images

Reporting box

Reporting on pericardial effusion

Summary

- Severity of effusion
- Evidence of cardiac tamponade

Qualitative data

- Apparent size of effusion: trace, small, moderate, large
- Global or loculated
- Site of maximal depth
- Evidence of fibrin strands or mass
- Evidence of diastolic atrial/right ventricular collapse
- Pattern of hepatic and pulmonary vein flow

Quantitative data

- Maximal depth
- Degree of respiratory variation at mitral/aortic valves

Reporting box

Reporting on pericardial constriction

Summary

- Diagnosis

Qualitative data

- Evidence of pericardial thickening
- Septal bounce
- Pattern of pulmonary and hepatic vein flow

Quantitative data

- Maximal pericardial thickness*
- E wave peak velocity
- E:A ratio
- Deceleration time
- E:e' ratio
- Degree of respiratory variation in transmitral/transtricuspid flow
- Inferior vena cava diameters/collapsibility

*Often unreliable.

Cardiac masses

Introduction

Intracardiac masses are rare echocardiographic findings. The differential diagnosis is quite broad, but can be narrowed down by basic characterisation according to location, size and appearance. The main categories of diagnosis are neoplasm, thrombus, vegetation, normal structure or artefact.

A definitive diagnosis cannot always be made from echo appearance alone, and sometimes a combination of clinical features, other imaging modalities and biopsy is required to reach a conclusion.

Primary neoplasms

Benign

Atrial myxoma

Atrial myxoma is the commonest primary cardiac neoplasm, but even so is a rare diagnosis. It almost always arises in the left atrium from the interatrial septum in the region of the fossa ovalis, but can arise from any cardiac chamber or even the mitral or tricuspid valves. They are usually solitary, though multiple myxomas occur in familial cases. Occasionally recurrence occurs after surgical removal.

Atrial myxoma can cause valvular obstruction due to tumour prolapsing through the mitral valve (Fig. 18.1). In addition, emboli can occur, due to either tumour breaking off or thrombus formation on the tumour.

The appearance of a myxoma needs to be distinguished from a large atrial thrombus (see Fig. 18.6, below). Classically, myxoma is attached to the interatrial septum and has a heterogeneous texture, often with evidence of cavitation

Figure 18.1

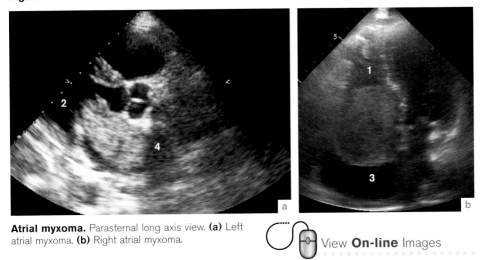

Atrial myxoma. Parasternal long axis view. **(a)** Left atrial myxoma. **(b)** Right atrial myxoma.

View **On-line** Images

Figure 18.2

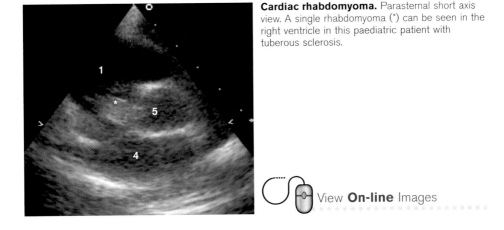

Cardiac rhabdomyoma. Parasternal short axis view. A single rhabdomyoma (*) can be seen in the right ventricle in this paediatric patient with tuberous sclerosis.

View **On-line** Images

(Fig. 18.1). In contrast, thrombus more commonly arises in the left atrial appendage and is homogeneous.

Cardiac rhabdomyoma

This is actually a non-neoplastic disorder (hamartoma) of striated muscle growth. Most cases occur in children and are associated with tuberous sclerosis. They arise anywhere in the heart (intramural or intracavitary) and are often multiple. The effects of the tumour on cardiac function depend on size and location (e.g. arrhythmia, valve obstruction). The echocardiographic features are usually of small, homogeneous, lobulated, hyperechoic tumours (Fig. 18.2).

Figure 18.3

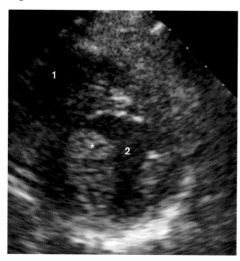

Cardiac metastasis. Parasternal short axis view. This patient was known to have advanced breast carcinoma. The interventricular septum appears thickened due to growth of a mass (*) which has distinct echo texture compared to the rest of the myocardium.

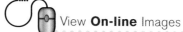
View **On-line** Images

Malignant

The commonest primary malignancies of the heart are sarcomas, and these usually arise in the right ventricle. They may be diffusely infiltrative, or discrete polypoid/sessile masses that extend into the pericardium/ventricular cavity. Distant metastases are usually present, and the prognosis is very poor.

Secondary neoplasms

Spread of tumour to the heart from other primary sites (metastases) is much more common than primary cardiac neoplasms. The commonest sites of origin include lung, breast, melanoma and lymphoma. Spread is either via the blood, or directly through the pericardium, and tumour deposits may involve any structure in the heart. The echocardiographic texture of the tumour is often distinct to surrounding cardiac muscle (Fig. 18.3).

Renal cell carcinoma is a special case of metastatic spread to the heart. It characteristically invades the renal vein and inferior vena cava. In advanced cases the tumour ascends the inferior vena cava and reaches the right atrium or even further, causing obstructive and embolic complications (Fig. 18.4). It may resemble a right atrial myxoma.

Thrombus

Intracardiac thrombus is more likely to occur if there is stagnation of blood, abnormal/damaged endothelium or abnormal coagulation. In the absence of predisposing factors for thrombus formation, alternative diagnoses should be considered.

The appearance of thrombus varies widely. It may be globular/pedunculated and mobile (Fig. 18.5a), or else laminated, immobile and echo-dense (Fig. 18.5c).

Figure 18.4

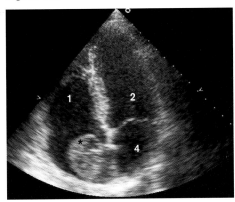

Renal cell carcinoma. Apical four-chamber view. A heterogeneous mass (*) can be seen occupying the right atrium. From this view it is not possible to distinguish the appearance from a right atrial myxoma (compare Fig. 18.1b). Further imaging and surgical resection confirmed a renal cell carcinoma.

View **On-line** Images

Figure 18.5

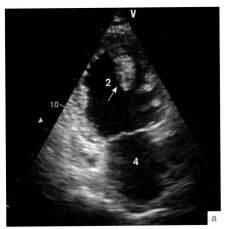

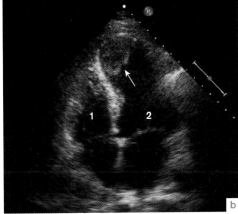

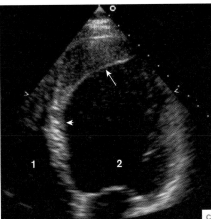

Left ventricular thrombus. (a) Apical two-chamber view. **(b** and **c)** Apical four-chamber view. **(a)** A large pedunculated thrombus (*) is seen in the left ventricular apex. The patient has a dilated cardiomyopathy. **(b)** Fresh apical mural thrombus following an anterior myocardial infarct (arrow). **(c)** Chronic laminated thrombus (arrow) following a remote history of myocardial infarction. It is of similar texture and thickness to the adjacent myocardium (arrowhead).

View **On-line** Images

Figure 18.6

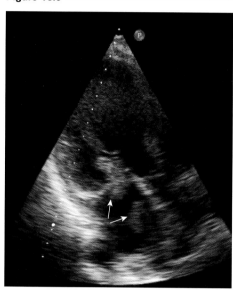

Left atrial thrombus. Apical three-chamber view. Two thrombi (arrows) are present in left atrium: one is attached to the mitral valve and the other has a septal attachment. The patient has atrial fibrillation and severe left ventricular dysfunction.

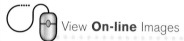
View **On-line** Images

Dilated cardiomyopathy and recent transmural myocardial infarction can be associated with mural thrombus at sites of akinesis. In this situation laminated thrombus can be mistaken for akinetic myocardium.

Atrial fibrillation and mitral stenosis characteristically lead to thrombus formation in the left atrial appendage, though other sites in the left atrium can be affected (Fig. 18.6). Transoesophageal echocardiography examination is required if definitive exclusion of left atrial thrombus is required.

Valvular masses

Infective endocarditis

The characteristics of vegetations and the differential diagnosis of valvular masses are discussed in Chapter 15.

Papillary fibroelastoma

This is a benign tumour affecting cardiac valves. Presentation is typically in middle to late adulthood with embolic complications such as stroke, or myocardial infarction. They are more common in the aortic and mitral valves and often occur on the 'downstream' side of the valve (e.g. ventricular side of the mitral valve). They have a characteristic frond-like appearance which has been likened to a sea anemone (Fig. 18.7).

Figure 18.7

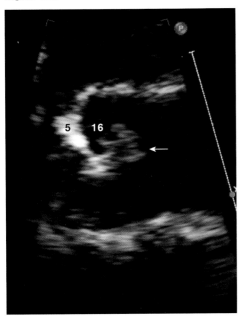

Papillary fibroelastoma. Magnified parasternal long axis view. There is a frond-like growth on the end of a stalk on the non-coronary cusp of the aortic valve (arrow): this was confirmed to be a papillary fibroelastoma after surgical resection.

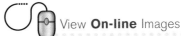 View **On-line** Images

Intravascular devices

Permanent pacemaker/implantable cardioverter defibrillator leads can often be seen in the right side of the heart as highly echogenic, thin, linear structures, but usually only a small portion is visualised at once so the appearance may initially be confusing (Fig. 18.8). Sometimes reverberation artefact is seen. Pacing leads may also be seen in the coronary sinus of patients with biventricular pacemakers for heart failure.

Devices are also used for closure of atrial and ventricular septal defects. These are structurally like an umbrella, with metallic struts radiating from the centre of the device, which is deployed flat against the septum. The final appearance is rather like a rivet (Fig. 18.9 and Fig. 20.11).

Normal variants and artefact

Normal variants, such as eustachian valve, moderator bands, lipomatous hypertrophy and Chiari networks, can be confused for other intracardiac masses. These are discussed in other chapters.

Echo artefacts arise for a variety of reasons, such as reverberation from echogenic structures (e.g. calcification, metallic structures). They tend not to conform to anatomical structures or boundaries, and are usually only seen from one echo window.

Figure 18.8

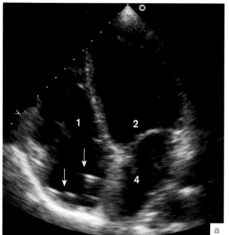
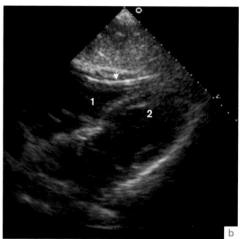
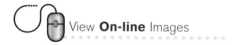

Pacing leads. (a) Apical four-chamber view: right atrial pacing lead (arrows). **(b)** Subcostal view: right ventricular pacing lead (arrowhead), with the tip positioned at the apex.

View **On-line** Images

Figure 18.9

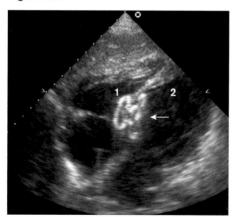

Ventricular septal defect closure device. Apical four-chamber view. The arrow indicates the position of a ventricular septal defect closure device.

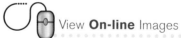

View **On-line** Images

Reporting box

Reporting on intracardiac masses

Summary

- Diagnosis or differential diagnosis
- Location
- Complications, e.g. valvular obstruction

Qualitative data

- Location of mass: luminal, valvular, mural, intramural, extracardiac
- Morphology: sessile, pedunculated
- Mobility: fixed, independent, tethered
- Echotexture: homogeneous, heterogeneous, cavitated, calcified, fluid-filled

Quantitative data

- Dimensions

The aorta

Introduction

Basic anatomy

The aorta is the main arterial conduit of the body and is divided into thoracic and abdominal portions by the diaphragm. The thoracic aorta is subdivided into ascending, arch and descending portions by the innominate and left subclavian arteries, respectively. The aortic arch therefore gives off all the major vessels to the head and upper limbs (Fig. 19.1). The aortic root includes the aortic annulus, the sinuses of Valsalva and the sinotubular junction.

The course of the thoracic aorta starts in the anterior mediastinum, within the pericardium to the right of the midline. It curves in front of the trachea, arching across to the left, and reaches the posterior mediastinum, where it lies in front of the thoracic vertebrae and behind the oesophagus.

Like all arteries, it is made up of three histologically distinct layers: the intima, media and adventitia. The intima is the thin inner layer of endothelium and subendothelial connective tissue. The media is a thick muscular layer that provides the majority of strength and elasticity. Finally, the adventitia is a fibrous protective outer layer.

Echocardiographic appearance

The aorta appears as a thin echo-bright tube. It is of uniform dimensions, except at the sinuses of Valsalva, where it is slightly dilated. The aortic root and proximal ascending aorta are usually seen on the parasternal long axis (PSLAX) view (Fig. 19.2). Part of the descending thoracic aorta is also seen behind the left atrium in this view. The right parasternal view is used to image the ascending aorta, whilst the suprasternal

Figure 19.1

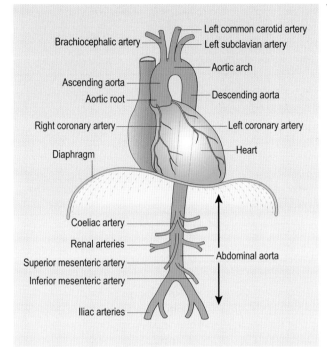

Brachiocephalic artery
Left common carotid artery
Left subclavian artery
Aortic arch
Ascending aorta
Aortic root
Descending aorta
Right coronary artery
Left coronary artery
Heart
Diaphragm
Coeliac artery
Renal arteries
Abdominal aorta
Superior mesenteric artery
Inferior mesenteric artery
Iliac arteries

The anatomy of the aorta.

Figure 19.2

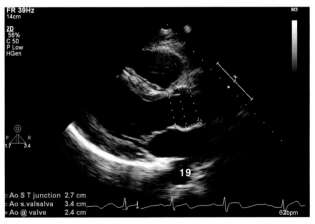

FR 39Hz
14cm

2D
56%
C 50
P Low
HGen

P   R
1.7   3.4

19

Ao S T junction 2.7 cm
Ao s.valsalva   3.4 cm
Ao @ valve   2.4 cm
62bpm

**Normal aortic root and
ascending aorta.** Parasternal
long axis view. The aortic root,
sinuses of Valsalva, sinotubular
junction and proximal ascending
aorta are seen. A portion of the
descending thoracic aorta is also
visualised behind the left atrium.

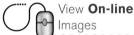

View **On-line**
Images

windows demonstrate the aortic arch and its branches (Fig. 19.3). The subcostal
window can be used to assess the suprarenal abdominal aorta.

Visualisation of the thoracic aorta with transthoracic echocardiography (TTE)
varies between patients. More often than not, images are suboptimal and it is not
possible to diagnose or exclude aortic pathology with certainty. Therefore if aortic

Figure 19.3

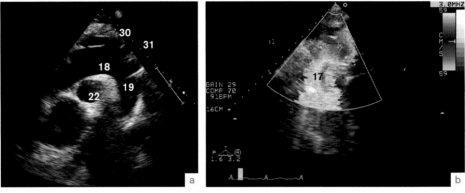

Normal aortic arch. Suprasternal views.
(a) Aortic arch and descending aorta.
(b) Ascending aorta (colour flow mapping Doppler).

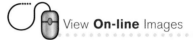 View **On-line** Images

pathology is suspected, other forms of imaging, such as transoesophageal echo (TOE), computed tomography (CT) or magnetic resonance imaging (MRI), are usually required to reach a firm diagnosis.

Standard measurements

The aortic root dimensions should be measured in every study. Measurements should be made at the aortic annulus (between the hinge points of the valve cusps), sinus of Valsalva and sinotubular junction (Fig. 19.2). Traditionally this has been done using M-mode in the PSLAX view, but this tends to underestimate the diameter, and direct measurements from two-dimensional images are now recommended. Normal values vary with body size and gender, and are given in Appendix 1. A useful rule of thumb is that the aortic root and proximal aorta should always be less than 3.7 cm in an average-sized adult. Indexing to body surface area should be reported routinely (see Appendix 1).

Diseases of the aorta

Aortic atheroma

Atherosclerosis can affect the aorta, like other major arteries, and often coexists with coronary atherosclerotic disease. Atheroma appears as a thickening of the arterial wall, which can be focal or generalised, and may be associated with calcification. Severe atheroma (>4 mm thick) or complex disease such as protruding or mobile atherosclerosis can be a cause of stroke and systemic embolism. Detection is far more reliable with TOE than TTE.

Thoracic aortic aneurysm

An aneurysm is a fixed localised dilatation of the aorta, which has a maximum diameter exceeding the upper limit of normal by 50%. Aneurysms may be fusiform (symmetrical dilatation) or saccular (asymmetrical, narrow-necked like a sac). Aneurysms are caused by diseases that either weaken the aortic wall or cause increased wall stress (Table 19.1).

Ascending aortic aneurysms tend to be caused by diseases that cause cystic necrosis of the media. This is particularly associated with Marfan's syndrome and other hereditary aortic syndromes, but can also occur with ageing and hypertension. Descending aneurysms are more frequently due to atherosclerosis.

Table 19.1 Causes of aortic aneurysm

Weakened wall

Atherosclerosis

Aortitis

Takayasu's arteritis

Ankylosing spondylitis and other spondyloarthritides

Giant cell arteritis

Collagen disorders

Marfan's syndrome

Ehlers–Danlos syndrome

Infection

Syphilis

Tuberculosis

Salmonella

Post-traumatic

Deceleration injuries

Catheter injury

Increased wall stress

Hypertension

Post aortic stenosis

Bicuspid aortic valve

Aortic coarctation

Figure 19.4

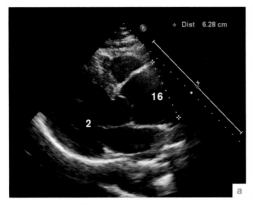

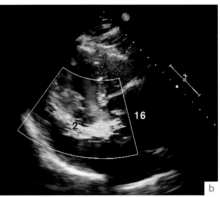

Ascending aortic aneurysm. Parasternal long axis view. **(a)** This patient has Marfan's syndrome. The aortic root and ascending aorta are severely dilated. **(b)** Aortic regurgitation secondary to aortic root dilatation.

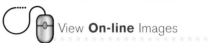 View **On-line** Images

Echocardiographic appearance

TTE (PSLAX view) is useful for detecting ascending aortic aneurysms, particularly those involving the aortic root and sinotubular junction, but is less reliable at identifying aneurysm at other sites. The echocardiographic appearance of an aneurysm is a region of dilatation (Fig. 19.4) that expands in systole. The maximal internal diameter should be measured and referenced to the patient's age and body surface area. The underlying cause may sometimes be deduced either from the characteristic appearance of the aneurysm (e.g. aortic root dilatation in Marfan's syndrome) or identification of other pathology (e.g. bicuspid aortic valve, coarctation). Dilatation of the aortic root can disrupt the aortic valve leaflets, causing aortic regurgitation (Fig. 19.4).

Elective surgical replacement of the ascending aorta is considered when the diameter exceeds 5.5 cm (4.5 cm in Marfan's syndrome), as the risk of spontaneous rupture is high.

Aortic dissection

Aortic dissection is a condition in which the intima shears apart from the rest of the aortic wall, forming a flap of tissue and a false lumen (Fig. 19.5). The dissection can propagate along the aortic wall and re-enter the true lumen at a distal site, or else cause occlusion of the aorta and its branches. When the aortic root is involved, acute severe aortic regurgitation, coronary artery occlusion and pericardial effusion can occur. Rupture into a pleural space occasionally occurs.

The underlying causes mirror those of aortic aneurysm, and it is particularly associated with conditions causing cystic medial necrosis.

Aortic dissection can be rapidly fatal and urgent treatment is warranted. Management is determined by the site of the dissection: involvement of the ascending aorta or arch (Stanford type A: Fig. 19.6) requires emergency aortic replacement,

Figure 19.5

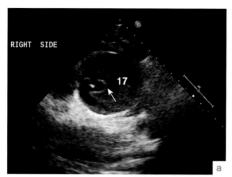
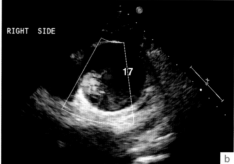

a

b

Dissection of the ascending aorta. Right parasternal view. **(a)** The dissection flap (arrow) is clearly seen separating the small true lumen and the larger false lumen. Note the spontaneous echo contrast in the false lumen. **(b)** Colour flow mapping demonstrates blood flow in the true lumen.

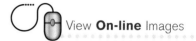 View **On-line** Images

Figure 19.6

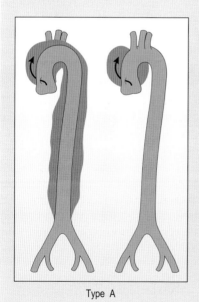

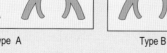

Type A   Type B

Classification of aortic dissection/intramural haematoma. Stanford classification. Type A: any involvement of the ascending aorta. Type B: restricted to the descending aorta.

whilst involvement confined to the descending thoracic aorta (type B) is treated by aggressive blood pressure lowering.

Echocardiographic appearance

Unequivocal echocardiographic evidence of aortic dissection requires demonstration of a mobile dissection flap, a false lumen and an entry or exit point between

Figure 19.7

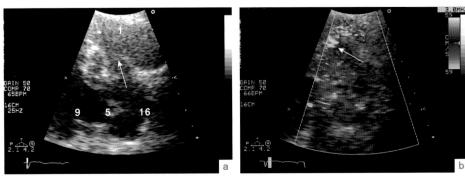

Ruptured sinus of Valsalva aneurysm. (a) The right
coronary sinus of Valsalva is aneurysmal (arrow).
(b) Doppler colour flow mapping demonstrates flow
between the coronary sinus and the right ventricle (arrow).

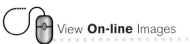
View **On-line** Images

the true and false lumens (Fig. 19.5). Most of the time, however, the findings on
TTE are more ambiguous, such as aortic root dilatation, acute aortic regurgitation,
aortic valve cusp prolapse, pericardial effusion and pleural effusion. Dissection
may also involve the coronary arteries, causing acute myocardial infarction, with
evidence of regional wall motion abnormalities. Definitive diagnosis usually
requires TOE, or else tomographic imaging (CT, MRI).

Sinus of Valsalva aneurysm

The sinuses of Valsalva are outpouchings of the aorta at the level of the aortic
valve cusps, from which the coronary arteries arise. They are not usually seen very
well on TTE.

Aneurysmal dilatation of the sinuses occurs most commonly as a congenital
condition, associated with ventricular septal defect. It can also develop in patients
with aortic root pathology, and following cardiac surgery. A rare complication
is aneurysm rupture, which usually causes aortic regurgitation into the right ventricle (Fig. 19.7), or other cardiac chamber, depending on the specific sinus involved.

Congenital aortic disease

Aortic coarctation

This is a constriction of the aorta due to abnormal embryonic development. It is
localised to the descending thoracic aorta distal to the origin of the left subclavian
artery, near the ligamentum arteriosus. It can occur in isolation, or associated with
other congenital defects, most notably bicuspid aortic valve. It has a particular
association with Turner's syndrome. The majority of cases are detected in infants,
but rare cases may present in adulthood with complications such as hypertension,
aortic dissection, aortic aneurysm, infective endocarditis, heart failure and cerebral
haemorrhage.

Figure 19.8

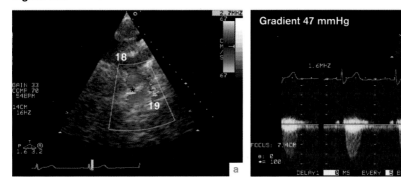
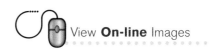

Aortic coarctation. (a) There is a ridge-like narrowing (*) in the descending thoracic aorta, associated with acceleration of blood flow on colour flow mapping (CFM: red jet on CFM Doppler). This appearance is suggestive of aortic coarctation. **(b)** Continuous wave Doppler across the coarctation estimates a gradient of 47 mmHg.

View **On-line** Images

Figure 19.9

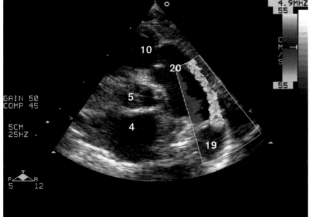

Patent ductus arteriosus.
Parasternal short axis view. There is blood flow from the descending thoracic aorta to the pulmonary artery, suggesting the presence of a patent ductus arteriosus.

View **On-line** Images

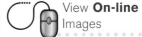

On a suprasternal view the coarctation appears as a ridge-like narrowing of the descending thoracic aorta, associated with turbulent high-velocity flow (Fig. 19.8). Less frequently a long tubular constriction occurs. Continuous wave Doppler is used to assess the severity of the gradient across the coarctation, using the Bernoulli equation. A gradient greater than 25 mmHg is considered severe enough to warrant intervention, either by surgery or percutaneous balloon dilatation. Such patients require echocardiographic follow-up to detect restenosis.

Patent ductus arteriosus

The ductus arteriosus is part of the fetal circulation, and connects the aorta to the pulmonary artery to supply the developing lungs with oxygenated blood *in utero*.

After birth it closes spontaneously in the majority of people, and fibroses to form the ligamentum arteriosum. It is frequently associated with other congenital abnormalities and is invariably detected and treated in infancy or childhood.

A patent ductus arteriosus can be seen best on the parasternal short axis view at the level of the right ventricular outflow tract using colour flow mapping. It appears as an abnormal jet of blood flow from the descending aorta to the pulmonary artery (Fig. 19.9). The pulmonary arteries may be dilated as a result of the high-pressure shunt.

Congenital septal abnormalities

Atrial septal defects

Embryology

During development the interatrial septum (IAS) is formed by the fusion of several different ridges of tissue. One part grows down from the upper part of the atria (septum primum), and the other grows up from the region of the primitive atrioventricular junction, known as the endocardial cushions. Holes form between the septa at various times in development and atrial septal defects (ASDs) are essentially a failure of these holes to close, or else complete failure of one part of the septum to grow.

Patent foramen ovale (PFO) and atrial septal aneurysm (ASA)

Normal fetal circulation relies on a communication between the right and left atria (foramen ovale) to divert oxygenated blood away from the lungs to the systemic circulation. Spontaneous closure of the foramen ovale occurs after birth in the majority of people, but it remains patent in up to 20% of adults. A PFO is always less than 5 mm in diameter.

On echo a PFO is suggested by an area of 'drop out' in the IAS, but this is a relatively non-specific finding, as the foramen ovale is usually thinner and less echo-dense than the rest of the septum, even if it is closed. The subcostal view is usually the best as the IAS is perpendicular to the ultrasound beam. Evidence of blood flow between the atria may be seen on colour flow mapping (CFM: Fig. 20.1), but failure to demonstrate this does not exclude a PFO. PFOs are often covered by a flap of tissue, so that under normal circumstances there is no shunt between the atria: if right atrial pressure is

Figure 20.1

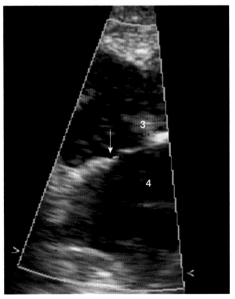

Patent foramen ovale. Colour flow mapping (CFM) subcostal view. The tiny trace of blood flow picked up on CFM (arrow) suggests the presence of a patent foramen ovale. This is best appreciated on the moving images.

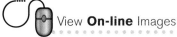

View **On-line** Images

increased (e.g. in the Valsalva manoeuvre), the flap may be displaced and a shunt occurs.

An ASA is an abnormality associated with PFO, but can occur in isolation: it is recognised by a region of hypermobile IAS that flops from side to side. If the pressure in one atrium or other is raised it may form a permanent bulge in the IAS. The strict definition for an ASA requires at least 1 cm excursion and a length of at least 1 cm (Fig. 20.2).

Bubble contrast studies

The most reliable test for a PFO is a bubble study using agitated saline as a contrast agent. Normal saline (9 ml) is agitated by rapidly mixing with ≤1 ml of air using two 10-ml syringes connected via a three-way tap. This is immediately injected into an arm vein whilst a long loop of echo images (about 10 seconds) is recorded from the apical four-chamber (A4C) or subcostal view. Clearly this technique requires two people for it to be performed successfully.

Microbubbles opacify the right heart, but under normal circumstances none should be seen in the left side of the heart because they are dissipated by the pulmonary capillaries. The presence of bubbles in the left atrium/ventricle suggests the presence of a right-to-left shunt, which may be at the level of the atria, ventricles or pulmonary circulation. A cardiac shunt is suggested by the appearance of bubbles in the left heart within four cardiac cycles of their presence in the right heart: longer delays suggest a pulmonary shunt.

A large PFO is defined by the presence of more than 20 microbubbles in the left side of the heart (Fig. 20.3). If there is no evidence of a shunt during normal respiration the Valsalva manoeuvre should be performed. Ask the patient to 'bear

Figure 20.2

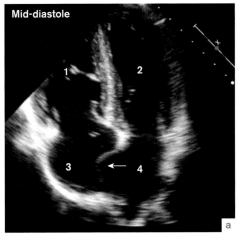

Mid-diastole

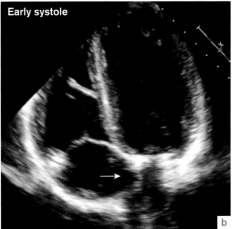

Early systole

Atrial septal aneurysm. (a and **b)** Apical four-chamber views. The interatrial septum has redundant tissue that is abnormally mobile (arrow), suggestive of an atrial septal aneurysm. A prominent Chiari network is also visible in the right atrium on the web image.

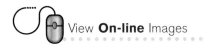

View **On-line** Images

Figure 20.3

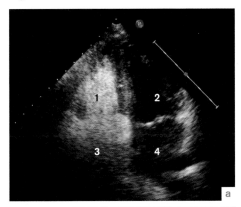

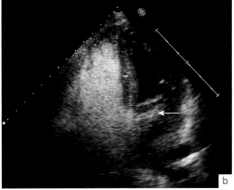

Intravenous bubble contrast study with Valsalva manoeuvre. Apical four-chamber views. **(a)** Strain phase of Valsalva manoeuvre. No visible shunt. **(b)** Release phase of Valsalva. A jet of bubbles crosses the IAS (arrow). **(c)** Complete opacification of the left sided chambers.

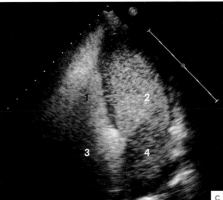

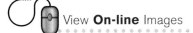

View **On-line** Images

down' as though straining on the toilet, and then breathe normally. This initially raises intrathoracic pressure, including the pressure in both atria, but also reduces venous return. When the strain is released, venous return increases, making right atrial pressure transiently increase above left atrial pressure. This pressure difference may be sufficient to force open the PFO flap, allowing a shunt of blood and microbubbles. Obtaining a good-quality echo during this can be difficult and a few practice runs should be tried before injecting contrast.

A negative transthoracic bubble contrast study cannot completely rule out a PFO and a transoesophageal echocardiography (TOE: with contrast/Valsalva) should be performed if necessary. In addition, injection of contrast from the femoral vein may be more sensitive than injection from the arm, since blood flow from the inferior vena cava is directed toward the foramen ovale by the eustachian valve.

Clinical syndromes associated with PFO

Cryptogenic stroke

The clinical significance of a PFO is controversial because it is such a common finding in the healthy population. Evidence suggests an association between PFO and cryptogenic stroke in young patients due to paradoxical emboli. The combination of PFO with an ASA is considered to predispose to stroke more strongly than a PFO alone. Device closure is considered in some patients, although recent trials have failed to demonstrate benefit.

Platypnoea orthodeoxia

This is a rare syndrome that presents in adulthood. It manifests as breathlessness and desaturation on sitting or standing up, with recovery lying flat. It is caused by profound right-to-left shunting of desaturated blood across a PFO (or secundum ASD). For reasons that are poorly understood, this is dependent on position and is therefore intermittent. Performing a TTE in a recumbent position may detect a PFO with left-to-right flow. Shunt reversal can be detected if the patient is scanned in a more upright position. However, without a high degree of suspicion the significance of a seemingly innocuous PFO may be easily overlooked.

Secundum atrial septal defect

Secundum ASD occurs as a result of either deficient growth of the septum secundum or resorption of the septum primum. It may be single, multiple or fenestrated, and can occur in isolation or associated with other congenital abnormalities. In 10% of cases one or more of the pulmonary veins drains into the right atrium/coronary sinus (anomalous pulmonary venous drainage).

A secundum ASD usually appears as a distinct break in the central portion of the IAS, near the fossa ovalis (Fig. 20.4). A fenestrated ASD has a lattice of tissue across the ASD and multiple jets of blood flow can be seen on CFM. A secundum ASD always has a distinct rim of septum separating it from the atrioventricular valve region, which distinguishes it from a primum ASD. As with PFOs the subcostal view is usually best, but secundum ASDs may also be seen on A4C and parasternal short axis (PSSAX) views.

Figure 20.4

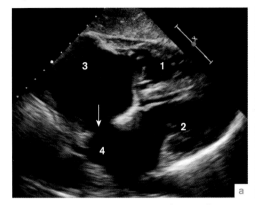
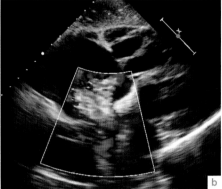

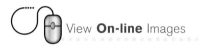

Secundum atrial septal defect. (a and **b)** Subcostal views. There is a 2-cm defect in the interatrial septum, characteristic of a secundum atrial septal defect. Colour flow mapping Doppler demonstrates a left-to-right shunt.

View **On-line** Images

Blood flow across the ASD can be demonstrated with Doppler techniques: flow is usually continuous, bidirectional but predominantly from left to right, and varies with respiration.

A large secundum ASD usually causes a significant left-to-right shunt, which may lead to right heart volume overload manifest as right ventricular dilatation and pulmonary hypertension. Right ventricular dilatation disproportionate to the size of the ASD suggests the possibility of anomalous pulmonary venous drainage. The size of a shunt can be estimated using quantitative pulse wave Doppler techniques to determine the systemic and pulmonary cardiac outputs (Qs and Qp) (see Chapter 11 and Fig. 20.10). Large shunts are usually apparent in childhood, whereas smaller shunts may not present until late adulthood.

A secundum ASD should be closed if the pulmonary flow is greater than twice that of the systemic flow (Qp:Qs >2:1). Closure can be performed surgically, but increasingly it is possible to use catheter-delivered devices (see Fig. 20.11).

Primum ASD

A primum ASD is caused by failed development of the endocardial cushions at the atrioventricular junction. It is a complex and severe defect that involves the central region of the heart where the atrial and ventricular septa meet the atrioventricular valves. In addition to an ASD, there may also be a ventricular septal defect (VSD), a cleft mitral valve or a common atrioventricular valve (Fig. 20.5). It usually presents in infancy and is often associated with Down's Syndrome.

Other ASDs

Two other types of ASD are recognised, but are very rare and difficult to visualise on transthoracic echo. Sinus venosus ASDs usually occur at the upper part of the

Figure 20.5

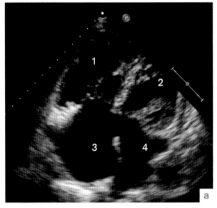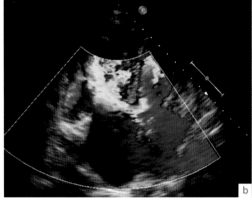

Primum atrial septal defect. (a and **b)** Apical four-chamber views. There is a defect in the interatrial septum adjacent to the atrioventricular valves and ventricular septum.

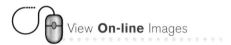
View **On-line** Images

IAS, where the superior vena cava enters the right atrium, so that the SVC effectively drains into both atria. More rarely they can occur in association with inferior vena cava. They are almost invariably associated with anomalous pulmonary venous drainage.

Coronary sinus ASDs occur in the region of the IAS adjacent to the coronary sinus, between the tricuspid annulus, inferior vena cava and eustachian ridge.

Ventricular septal defects

VSD is the commonest congenital cardiac abnormality in children. The interventricular septum is derived from a variety of embryological components, so that abnormal development of one or another can lead to distinct types of VSD. The terminology is confusing and simply has to be learned.

Conoventricular VSD (outlet VSD)

This is the commonest type (75%), arising in the region of the left and right ventricular outflow tracts, near the aortic and pulmonary valves. There are three different types: perimembranous, subpulmonic or misaligned.

Perimembranous VSD

A perimembranous VSD is located adjacent to the medial papillary muscle of the tricuspid valve. Characteristically, blood flow can be detected between the left ventricle and the right ventricular outflow tract (RVOT) at the 11 o'clock position in a PSSAX view at the level of the aortic valve (Fig. 20.6). Spontaneous closure

Figure 20.6

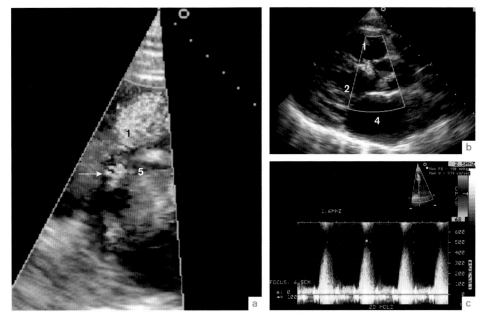

Perimembranous ventricular septal defect (VSD). **(a)** Parasternal short axis view. The VSD communicates with the right ventricle in the region of the aortic valve. Blood flow from left to right is indicated by colour flow mapping (arrow). **(b)** Parasternal long axis view. In this view the VSD is located just below the aortic valve. **(c)** Continuous wave Doppler demonstrates a peak gradient of 108 mmHg across the VSD.

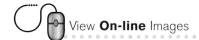 View **On-line** Images

can occur, incorporating part of the septal leaflet of the tricuspid valve, leaving an aneurysmal membrane (Fig. 20.7).

Subpulmonic VSD

A subpulmonic VSD is located adjacent to the pulmonary valve: on the PSSAX view it is located at the 1 o'clock position (Fig. 20.8).

Misaligned VSD

This occurs in tetralogy of Fallot and is invariably detected in childhood.

Muscular VSD

These can occur in any location within the mid or apical walls of the interventricular septum (Fig. 20.9). About 60% close spontaneously during childhood.

Figure 20.7

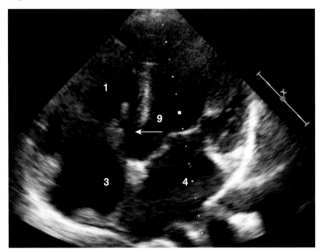

Perimembranous ventricular septal defect: spontaneous closure. Apical four-chamber view. Partial closure of a perimembranous VSD has occurred, incorporating part of the septal leaflet of the tricuspid valve (arrow).

View **On-line** Images

Figure 20.8

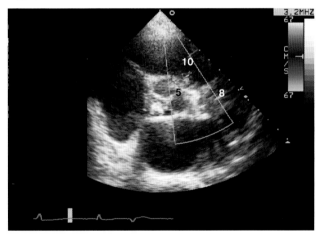

Subpulmonic ventricular septal defect. Parasternal short axis view. Colour flow mapping locates the VSD just before the pulmonary valve in the right ventricular outflow tract.

View **On-line** Images

Inlet VSD

Inlet VSDs are rare and are associated with primum ASD. They are located adjacent to the tricuspid valve and are usually associated with abnormalities of the atrioventricular valves (e.g. cleft mitral valve).

The significance of a VSD depends mainly on the size of shunt. A small shunt is unlikely to have any haemodynamic effect and can be managed conservatively. A large defect will cause a significant shunt from the high-pressure left ventricle to the low-pressure right ventricle. Although quantitative techniques can estimate the

Figure 20.9

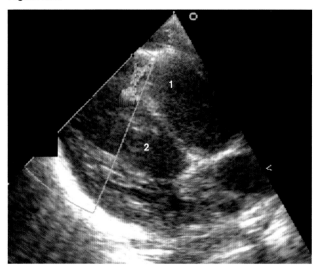

Muscular ventricular septal defect. Parasternal long axis view. In this case the VSD is located in the apical interventricular septum. Colour flow mapping detects a left-to-right shunt.

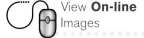

View **On-line** Images

size of the shunt, signs of right ventricular dilatation indicate that the shunt is likely to be large. Furthermore, the development of pulmonary hypertension may eventually lead to equalisation of the left and right ventricular pressures, and the volume of the shunt may become minimal.

Right ventricular systolic pressure (RVSP) can be estimated from the peak systolic velocity across the VSD using continuous wave Doppler (Fig. 20.6c). This allows the pressure difference between the ventricles to be calculated using the modified Bernoulli equation: since systolic blood pressure (SBP) is approximately equal to left ventricular systolic pressure (assuming no aortic stenosis), then RVSP is given from the following equation: RVSP (mmHg) = SBP – VSD pressure gradient.

Quantitative assessment of intracardiac shunts

An important part of the assessment of intracardiac shunts, such as atrial or VSDs, is quantification of the magnitude of the shunt by comparing the pulmonary (Qp) and systemic outputs (Qs) of the heart. The technique relies on the principles of the (dis)continuity equation described in Chapter 11. For example, if there is significant blood flow through a VSD from the left ventricle to the right ventricle, then right-sided cardiac output will exceed that of the left (Qp>Qs). Ventricular stroke volumes can be measured at the RVOT and left ventricular outflow tract, respectively, using the standard measures of velocity time integral and outflow tract diameters. A shunt ratio of 2:1 is considered significant. A worked example is given in Figure 20.10.

Figure 20.10

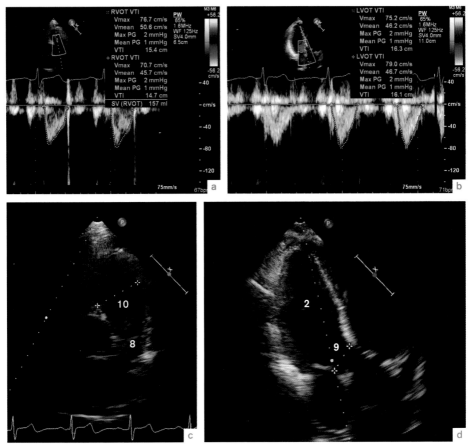

Quantitative assessment of an intracardiac shunt. The data is derived from the atrial septal defect case in Figure 20.4. **(a)** Pulse wave Doppler: right ventricular outflow tract (RVOT) velocity time integral (VTI) 15.1 cm. **(b)** Pulse wave Doppler left ventricular outflow tract (LVOT) VTI 16.2 cm. **(c)** Parasternal short axis view: RVOT diameter 3.6 cm. **(d)** Apical three-chamber: LVOT diameter 2.2 cm.
Left ventricular stroke volume = $3.142 \times 1.1^2 \times 16.2 = 62$ ml
Right ventricular stroke volume = $3.142 \times 1.8^2 \times 15.1 = 154$ ml
Therefore Qp:Qs = 154/62 = 2.5
This suggests a large shunt and is in keeping with the right heart dilatation.

Percutaneous device closure

Percutaneous closure of septal defects is an effective, minimally invasive option for the treatment of PFOs, secundum ASD and certain VSDs. A variety of devices are available which comprise two umbrella structures that clamp either side of the defect when fully deployed (Fig. 20.11). Full closure of the defect does not occur until the device has become endothelialised after several months.

Secundum ASD can be closed percutaneously as long as the defect is <4 cm, with a rim of at least 0.5 cm separating the ASD from the pulmonary and aortic valves. Contraindications include anomalous pulmonary venous drainage (a

Figure 20.11

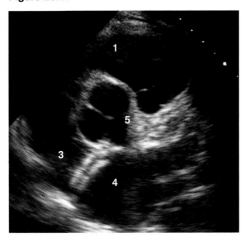

Patent foramen ovale closure device.
Parasternal short axis view. The closure device can be seen within the interatrial septum (arrow), and has the appearance of a button.

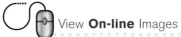

View **On-line** Images

TOE is required to exclude this), severe pulmonary hypertension, Eisenmenger's syndrome and other coexisting congenital cardiac defects requiring surgical correction.

Similar devices can be used to close muscular VSDs. Perimembranous VSDs, by virtue of their location near the pulmonary and aortic valves, are more difficult to close percutaneously.

Reporting box

Reporting on atrial septal defects

Summary

- Diagnosis
- Size of defect
- Shunt characteristics
- Associated lesions

Qualitative data

- Location of defect
- Shunt direction
- Associated lesions, e.g. anomalous pulmonary venous drainage
- Secondary remodelling, e.g. right heart dilatation, tricuspid regurgitation

Quantitative data

- Defect size
- Shunt ratio Qp:Qs
- Pulmonary artery pressure
- Atrial sizes
- Right ventricular dimensions
- Inferior vena cava diameter

Reporting box

Reporting on ventricular septal defects

Summary

- Diagnosis
- Shunt characteristics
- Associated lesions

Qualitative data

- Location and type of defect
- Shunt direction
- Associated lesions, e.g. atrial septal defect, valvular disease
- Secondary remodelling, e.g. right heart dilatation, tricuspid regurgitation

Quantitative data

- Size of defect
- Shunt ratio
- Shunt gradient
- Ventricular dimensions
- Pulmonary artery pressure

3D echocardiography

Introduction

The major development in echocardiography over the turn of the century has been the evolution and clinical utilisation of three-dimensional (3D) echocardiography. Available in both transthoracic and transoesophageal modalities, the use of 3D echocardiography has enhanced the accuracy of quantification and anatomical assessment. Teaching and training in echocardiography have also been improved by the ability to use 3D datasets to demonstrate the principles of standard two-dimensional (2D) imaging planes and relating echocardiographic images to standard anatomical projections.

Principles of 3D echo

Standard 2D echocardiography relies on a thin beam of ultrasound passing through tissue and the subsequent images derived from the reflected ultrasound beam. The technology involved in 3D echocardiography has now evolved to transducers densely packed with ultrasound crystals aligned and able to transmit and receive ultrasound on many scan lines, forming a pyramidal region of ultrasound interrogation, which is then rendered and shaded to form the impression of a 3D image on the screen.

Acquisition of a good 3D dataset relies on the same principles as 2D ultrasound, including:

- crisp electrocardiograph (ECG) trace – essential for generation of 'stitched' 3D volumes

- optimised window – breath hold for stable image position
- optimised controls – depth, focus, gain and sector width adjusted.

As 3D transducers contain more electronic circuitry and cabling than 2D transducers they are heavier and have a slightly larger footprint – this increases the need to work hard at finding an optimum window and contact point for a clean artefact-free acquisition. Furthermore, as the basic speed of ultrasound through tissue cannot be overcome, achieving adequate frame rates with 3D imaging can be difficult, emphasising the need to optimise machine settings as much as possible.

There are five different modes of 3D acquisition available with current platforms, and these are summarised in Table 21.1 (Figs 21.1 and 21.2).

Figure 21.1

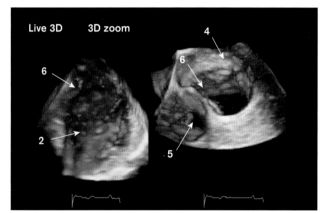

A comparison of live three-dimensional (3D) transoesophageal echocardiography (TOE) and 3D zoom TOE imaging of a mitral valve.

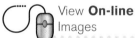
View **On-line** Images

Figure 21.2

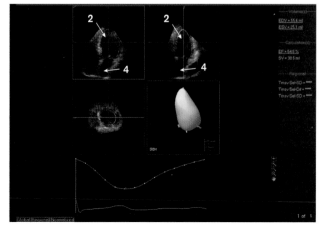

A full-volume acquisition over 4 beats of the whole left ventricle and semiautomated ejection fraction analysis.

Table 21.1 Three-dimensional (3D) echo modes

Modes	Comment	Frame rate	Limitations	Advantage	Main use
Live 3D	Single thin pyramidal volume	Good – usually > 30 Hz	Volume not wide enough to encompass whole of structures such as mitral valve	High frame rate and true live imaging	Limited clinical use
3D zoom	User-defined volume of interest	Depends on size of volume – typically 5–20 Hz	Frame rates low with wide volumes	True live imaging and can encompass whole structure	Mitral valve imaging, guiding interventions
Full volume	ECG-gated stitching of multiple pyramidal volumes to produce a large 3D volume	Depends on heart rate and depth, but usually >25 Hz	Requires regular rhythm and stable position to avoid stitching artefacts, not true live imaging	Generates high-resolution datasets	3D assessment of left ventricular size and function
3D colour	Available on live 3D and full-volume modes	Poor – even with small volumes frame rate often <10 Hz	Achieving adequate frame rates is at expense of volume size	Small colour jets can be displayed very well	3D quantification of mitral regurgitation inflow, paravalvular leaks
X-plane	Real-time imaging in two orthogonal planes	Good – usually >30 Hz	Not 3D imaging as two 2D imaging planes projected side by side	Excellent frame rates and aids rapid assessment of pathology and anatomy	Understanding anatomy of structures and identification of artefacts

ECG, electrocardiograph; 2D, two-dimensional.

Imaging protocol

Transthoracic 3D echocardiography

Technically a 3D dataset can be generated from any imaging window, but in practice the main use of routine 3D echocardiography is to enhance the accuracy of left ventricular (LV) volume and function assessment. The steps to achieve an ECG-gated 3D full volume of the LV are as follows (Fig. 21.3):

1. Ensure crisp ECG with good R-wave triggering.
2. Start in standard apical four-chamber (A4C) position with 2D imaging.
3. Optimise depth, 2D gain and sector width for 2D image.
4. Assess effect of respiration and likely duration of acquisition (usually four R-R cycles).
5. Select 'full-volume' acquisition.
6. Ensure 'biplane' imaging display mode is active.
7. Suspend respiration when both four-chamber and two-chamber views are optimised.
8. Start 'full-volume' acquisition – ensure patient, probe and ECG signal are stable.
9. Restart respiration.

Figure 21.3

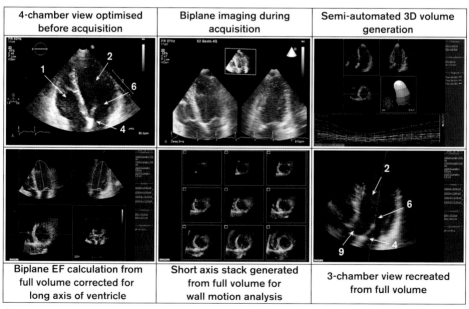

4-chamber view optimised before acquisition	Biplane imaging during acquisition	Semi-automated 3D volume generation
Biplane EF calculation from full volume corrected for long axis of ventricle	Short axis stack generated from full volume for wall motion analysis	3-chamber view recreated from full volume

(a–f) Steps in acquiring a transthoracic full-volume image. 3D, three-dimensional; EF, ejection fraction.

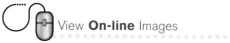 View **On-line** Images

10. Review acquisition for ECG regularity and triggering and stitching artefacts.

11. Store 3D volume if acceptable for subsequent analysis.

From a single 3D dataset acquired from the A4C position it is possible to 'generate' equivalent images of the 2D A4C, apical two-chamber (A2C), apical three-chamber (A3C) and apical five-chamber (A5C) views by appropriate cropping and manipulation of the pyramidal volume. Additional crops to 'isolate' the mitral, aortic and tricuspid valves are also possible.

A major advantage of the pyramidal volume is that the whole of the LV is captured, and any foreshortening evident in a standard 2D view can be corrected by aligning a cropping plane with the true cardiac apex. This is the principal reason behind the increased accuracy of LV volume assessment with 3D dataset analysis.

Transoesophageal echocardiography (TOE)

The most robust use of 3D TOE has been in the assessment and understanding of mitral valve pathology, in particular the ability to generate a 'surgeon's view' of the mitral valve to guide planning for mitral valve repair and uniform description of valve anatomy and pathology. The best images of the mitral valve are generated using the 3D zoom modality (Fig. 21.4).

Figure 21.4

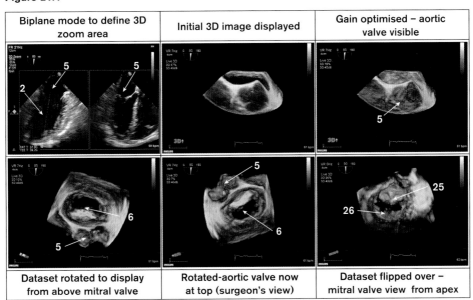

Biplane mode to define 3D zoom area	Initial 3D image displayed	Gain optimised – aortic valve visible
Dataset rotated to display from above mitral valve	Rotated-aortic valve now at top (surgeon's view)	Dataset flipped over – mitral valve view from apex

(a–f) Steps in acquiring a three-dimensional (3D) zoom transoesophageal echocardiography (TOE) acquisition of the mitral valve.

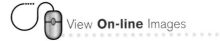 View **On-line** Images

1. Ensure stable 2D imaging window with clear view of mitral valve – usually at 0 or 90°.
2. Activate 3D zoom mode – a biplane image is generated.
3. Adjust box size and box position controls to cover mitral annulus on left-hand screen.
4. Adjust elevation width control to ensure sample box covers mitral annulus and leaflets on right-hand screen.
5. Ensure 3D zoom sample box is no larger than needed to cover mitral valve to ensure good frame rates.
6. Start 3D zoom acquisition proper.
   At this point an initially disappointing image will appear as the selected 3D volume will be projected from the side view and often with excessive gain. The mitral valve is held within this volume and in order to view it further steps are required:
7. Roll the 3D volume down to allow viewing from 'above'.
8. Reduce gain to eliminate blood pool noise (reducing too far will generate artefacts).
9. Rotate dataset around z-axis to position aortic valve at 12 o'clock.
10. Acquire 3D zoom volume or continue live imaging.

In practice the 3D zoom dataset can be acquired and stored after step 6 as all of the additional steps can be performed offline. However, when guiding interventions these steps are performed 'live' and the image is then updated continuously and will alter if the probe is moved.

Clinical applications

Assessment of left ventricular function

Evaluation of LV size and systolic function is the most important and common clinical reason for an echo study. Assessment of ventricular volume and mass by 2D is based on geometric assumptions. These assumptions render LV volume measurements inaccurate in patients with LV geometric distortions, such as regional wall motion abnormalities and cardiomyopathies. 3D echocardiographic techniques provide an advantage over the traditional methods, since they are not dependent on appropriate plane positioning or geometric assumptions (Table 21.2). As such, 3D echo is an excellent tool for the assessment of LV size, volume and function. Several studies have confirmed strong correlation of LV volumes calculated by 3D with the 'gold standard technique' of cardiac magnetic resonance.

The LV full volume is acquired from the A4C and A2C views on breath hold to minimise stitching artefacts. Recent studies have confirmed that a minimum of two heart beats is required for an adequate LV volume assessment.

The semiautomated software is used to identify landmarks and endocardial boundaries in the ventricle in systole and diastole. The accuracy of the endocardial border definition can be checked by scrolling through ventricular slices in the short axis. Using the defined endocardial borders, the software constructs a deformable

Table 21.2 Advantages and disadvantages of assessment of left ventricular (LV) function with three-dimensional (3D) echocardiography

Advantages	Allows for accurate assessment of an important and frequent clinical question
	Does not rely on geometric assumptions
	Avoids foreshortening of the LV
	Improved intraobserver and interobserver assessment
	Excellent correlation with cardiac MRI results for mass, ejection fraction and volumes
Disadvantages	Access to a 3D echo-capable machine and analysis software is required
	Multiple heart beat acquisitions are difficult with irregular heart beats
	Additional offline time is needed for manipulation of dataset

MRI, magnetic resonance imaging.

Figure 21.5

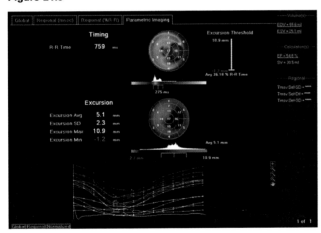

Segmental analysis of left ventricular function derived from a full-volume acquisition over 4 beats.

cast model of the LV. The LV systolic and diastolic volumes are calculated and an ejection fraction is obtained (Fig. 21.2). The LV cast model also allows for individual tracking and analysis of individual LV segments based on the 17-segment model (Fig. 21.5). This allows for objectively identifying wall motion abnormalities and measuring several LV segmental parameters.

Assessment of valvular heart disease

3D echocardiography, and in particular 3D TOE, has revolutionised imaging and understanding of valve anatomy and function, particularly the mitral valve, where

Figure 21.6

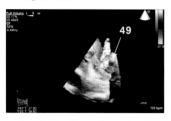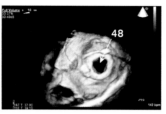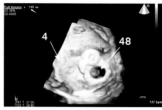

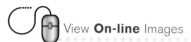

(a–c) Live three-dimensional (3D) transoesophageal echocardiography (TOE) imaging of a catheter intervention to close a paravalvular leak alongside a mechanical mitral valve.

View **On-line** Images

extraordinarily detailed and realistic renderings of the valve can be generated. This makes correct identification of prolapsed segments much easier and, by generating a surgeon's view of the valve, aids communication and surgical planning. Prosthetic mitral valves can also be imaged with great clarity to the point where individual sutures can be counted. Identification of pathology such as paravalvular leaks, thrombus formation and valve dysfunction is significantly easier with 3D imaging.

A full-volume dataset allows generation of any 2D imaging plane without constraint by the acoustic window. This has clear advantages in generation of a true orthogonal plane to a valve orifice – in mitral stenosis, for example. By ensuring the 2D plane is truly aligned to the leaflet tips and orthogonal to flow, increased accuracy of orifice planimetry is possible.

The aortic valve is more challenging to image in 3D as it is perpendicular to most standard TOE views and shielded to some extent by the aorta. 3D zoom and live 3D modes can be used to generate clear renderings of the aortic valve anatomy both from the aortic side and from underneath the aortic valve using a transgastric window.

Guiding interventions

An ever-increasing number of pathologies can now be treated with catheter-based approaches rather than cardiac surgery and these are frequently guided by echocardiography as well as traditional fluoroscopy. The advent of 3D echocardiography (particularly 3D TOE) has enhanced the ability of echocardiographers to assist in catheter placement, device deployment and procedural assessment (Fig. 21.6). When following catheters within cardiac chambers it is usually best to use 3D zoom mode if acceptable frame rates can be obtained, as it is a true live mode and the catheter's position will be rendered in real time.

Summary

3D echocardiography represents a significant advance in cardiac ultrasound technology and with modern platforms is relatively quick and simple to obtain. The principal benefit to standard transthoracic imaging is enhanced accuracy of quantification of LV size and function. 3D TOE has transformed the assessment of mitral valve disease, none more so than in the surgical planning environment. However, 3D echocardiography is not a panacea and cannot magically transform poor-quality 2D imaging. The need to concentrate on window and image optimisation is even more crucial to obtain useful and reproducible images.

Limitations

The cost of 3D echocardiography platforms has reduced considerably since their inception, as have the size and weight of the transducer probes. With enhanced acquisition modes, acquiring a 3D volume requires very few additional steps and little extra time and may indeed reduce the need for some 2D acquisitions. The principal limitations remain:

- Frame rate – balancing frame rates against volume size can be challenging.
- ECG gating – avoiding stitching artefacts in full-volume acquisitions can be difficult.
- Learning curve – obtaining the 3D datasets is straightforward but understanding how best to crop, align and display the images takes some practice.
- Heating – prolonged 3D TOE imaging increases probe heating of soft tissues.
- Workflow – increased offline analysis time is required for 3D volumetric assessment.

Future directions

3D transthoracic probes are rapidly approaching the size and shape of standard 2D transthoracic probes, allowing combined 2D and 3D imaging in one probe. Further miniaturisation and increased crystal density may improve resolution and frame rates. Development of standardised 3D protocols, nomenclature and image displays will help to increase uptake of 3D technology and integration into routine echocardiography practice.

The comprehensive examination

Integrating information

A comprehensive echo examination should be more than an exercise in technical competence. Before you even pick up the echo probe you need to familiarise yourself with the referral problem, and any other clinically relevant information about your patient. Useful information to bear in mind includes the suspected diagnosis or clinical problem, patient symptoms, clinical examination findings, past medical history, electrocardiograph and chest X-ray findings. Clearly there is some responsibility on the part of the referrer to provide detailed and accurate information.

Armed with this you should actively consider the possible diagnoses that need to be made, or excluded. For example, in a patient with peripheral oedema, it would be easy to miss evidence of constrictive pericarditis if you were not specifically thinking of this as a possible diagnosis.

As you perform the echo you should be seeking to clarify and refine your findings to reach a complete diagnosis: for example, if you find significant mitral regurgitation, further thought is required about the possible mechanism, the secondary effects and how you might look for evidence of this during the echo study.

The echo examination

Opinions differ as to what constitutes a comprehensive echo examination. In essence, you should use all appropriate modalities from every possible echo window, though some views and measurements are probably more important than others. In general it is best to stick to a standard routine, so that the maximum information is gathered with the minimum fuss. Obviously you may already have a routine that works for you, or you may need to be selective according to your patient's problem, the time available and your skill level.

As the examination progresses, you will keep encountering each structure from a different view, gathering further information that needs to be interpreted and added to what you have already discovered. Although it can be tempting to focus on one finding or structure, it is probably best to stick to a systematic approach that covers everything, and then integrate all the information at the end.

The series of echocardiographic views given in Table 22.1 should form the basis for a complete examination.

Table 22.1 The basis for a complete examination

| View | Assessment | | |
	2D imaging	Dimensions	Doppler
PSLAX			
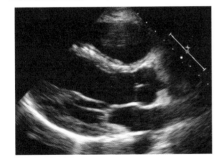	Aortic valve Mitral valve Left ventricle RV LA Pericardium	M-mode or B mode dimensions: Aortic root LA IVSd IVSs LVIDd LVIDs PWTd PWTs	Aortic and mitral valve: CFM Interventricular septum: CFM
RV inflow			
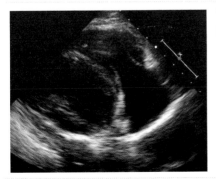	Tricuspid valve Right atrium		Tricuspid valve: CFM and CW

Table 22.1 *Continued*

View	Assessment		
	2D imaging	*Dimensions*	*Doppler*

RV outflow

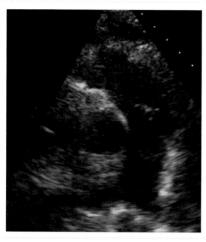

| | Pulmonary valve | RVOT diameter | Pulmonary valve: |
| | Pulmonary artery | Pulmonary artery diameter | CFM and CW RVOT: PW |

PSSAX: papillary level

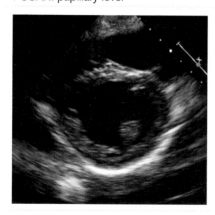

	Left ventricle	M-mode dimensions of left ventricle if not obtainable from PSLAX view	
	Right ventricle		
	Pericardium		

PSSAX: mitral level

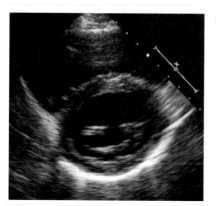

| | Mitral valve structure | | Mitral valve: CFM |

Table 22.1 *Continued*

View	Assessment		
	2D imaging	**Dimensions**	**Doppler**

PSSAX: aortic level

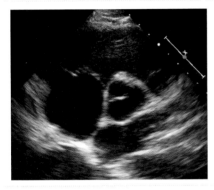

	Aortic valve	RVOT	Aortic valve:
	Tricuspid valve	diameter	CFM
	Pulmonary	Pulmonary	Tricuspid
	valve	artery	valve: CFM/
		diameter	CW/PW
			RVOT: PW
			Pulmonary
			valve: CFM/
			CW

A4C

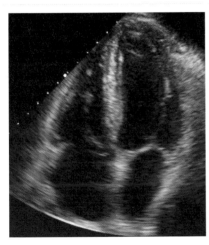

	LV	LV: volume in	Mitral valve:
	RV	systole and	CFM/PW/
	Interventricular	diastole	CW
	septum	(biplane EF)	Tricuspid
	Left atrium	RV dimensions	valve:
	Right atrium	RV area	CFM/PW/
	Interatrial	change	CW
	septum	LA volume	Pulmonary
	Pericardium	(biplane)	vein:
	Mitral valve	RA area	PW
	Tricuspid valve	LV MAPSE	IAS: CFM
		RV TAPSE	IVS: CFM
			Tissue
			Doppler:
			LV lateral and
			septal mitral
			annulus
			RV tricuspid
			annulus

Table 22.1 *Continued*

View	Assessment		
	2D imaging	**Dimensions**	**Doppler**
A5C			
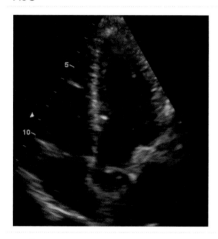	Aortic valve LVOT	LVOT diameter	Aortic valve: CFM and CW LVOT: PW
A2C			
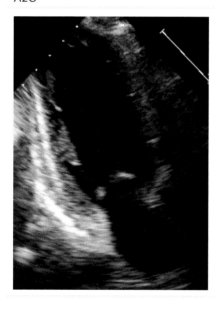	Left ventricle Mitral valve Left atrium Pericardium	LV: volume in systole and diastole (biplane EF) LA volume (biplane)	Mitral valve: CFM

Table 22.1 *Continued*

View	Assessment		
	2D imaging	**Dimensions**	**Doppler**

A3C

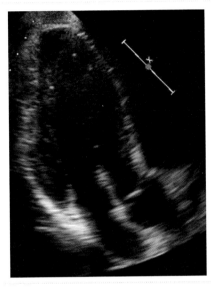

	2D imaging	Doppler
	Aortic valve	Aortic valve:
	Mitral valve	CFM ± CW
	LV	Mitral valve:
	LA	CFM
	Pericardium	

Subcostal 4C

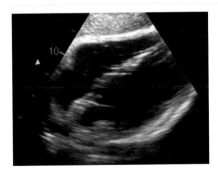

	2D imaging	Doppler
	LV	Mitral valve:
	RV	CFM
	Interventricular septum	Tricuspid valve:
	LA	CFM/CW
	RA	IAS: CFM
	Interatrial septum	IVS: CFM
	Pericardium	
	Mitral valve	
	Tricuspid valve	

Table 22.1 *Continued*

View	Assessment		
	2D imaging	*Dimensions*	*Doppler*

Subcostal IVC

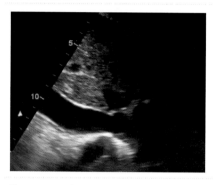

| | IVC collapsibility | IVC diameter | Hepatic vein: PW |

Suprasternal

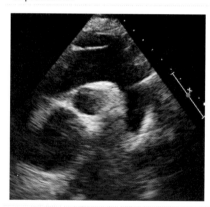

| | Aortic arch | Dimension of aortic arch | Aortic arch: CFM Descending aorta: PW and CW |

Right parasternal

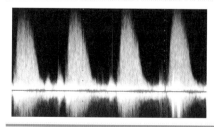

| | Ascending aortic structure | Ascending aortic dimension | Aortic valve: CW (Pedoff probe) |

The focused examination

Introduction

In an emergency situation, you may not want to perform a full echo examination, and you simply need to answer one or two specific questions. It is helpful to have an idea of what you are looking for and to concentrate on the relevant things: of course keep your eyes open for the unexpected. In such situations you may have minimal time, limited views and many people getting in the way. Remember that echo is not 100% reliable so you cannot exclude specific diagnoses with absolute certainty, but you may be able to make a diagnosis that is lifesaving. Also, bear in mind that you may come across incidental findings that are not likely to be directly relevant to the cause of the patient's deterioration and these should not be dwelt upon.

In the peri-arrest situation you need to examine quickly:

- left ventricular structure and function
- right ventricular structure and function
- pericardial effusion ± evidence of tamponade (e.g. right atrial/right ventricular diastolic collapse)
- valve structure and function: particularly evidence of critical aortic stenosis or acute severe mitral regurgitation on two-dimensional or colour flow mapping images
- pulmonary artery pressure
- inferior vena caval diameter.

In the following tables the differential diagnosis for each clinical situation has been restricted to conditions that can be detected by echo. The wider differential diagnosis is not considered, and many other causes may also be relevant. It is also important to note that echocardiography may not be the optimal diagnostic tool for all conditions listed, nor is it a substitute for clinical examination or acumen. However, as a readily available diagnostic tool a prompt focused echo study may be able to exclude significant cardiopulmonary disease in an acutely ill patient, allowing attention to be directed to diagnosing alternative causes.

Cardiac arrest (pulseless electrical activity)

Differential diagnosis	Echo findings
Cardiac tamponade	Pericardial effusion
	Myocardial rupture
Pulmonary embolism	Right ventricular dilatation/hypokinesia
Hypovolaemia/anaphylaxis	Inferior vena cava collapse/dynamic left ventricle
Tension pneumothorax	Unable to image heart

Acute chest pain

Differential diagnosis	Echo findings
Ischaemic heart disease	Regional wall motion abnormality
Pulmonary embolism	Right ventricular dilatation, pulmonary hypertension
Acute aortic syndromes*	Dissection flap, aortic aneurysm, atrial regurgitation, pericardial effusion
Pericarditis	Normal or pericardial effusion
Pneumonia	Pleural effusion ± consolidated lung
Outflow obstruction	Severe aortic stenosis or hypertrophic obstructive cardiomyopathy

*Best imaged by transoesophageal echocardiography.

Acute breathlessness

Differential diagnosis	Echo findings
Left ventricular failure	Left ventricular dysfunction
	Severe valvular heart disease
Pulmonary embolism	Right ventricular dilatation, pulmonary hypertension
Pneumonia	Consolidated lung base, pleural effusion
Pleural effusion	Pleural effusion

Hypotension

Differential diagnosis	Echo findings
Cardiogenic shock	Severe left ventricular dysfunction
	Severe right ventricular dysfunction
	Severe aortic stenosis
	Acute severe mitral regurgitation
	Ventricular septal defect post myocardial infarct
	Pericardial tamponade
Pulmonary embolism	Right ventricular dilatation, pulmonary hypertension
Hypovolaemia	Inferior vena cava collapse, hyperdynamic left ventricle

Ventricular arrhythmia

Differential diagnosis	Echo findings
Idiopathic	Normal
Ischaemic heart disease	Left ventricular dysfunction/regional wall motion abnormality
Dilated cardiomyopathy*	Left ventricular dysfunction
Valvular heart disease	Severe valvular dysfunction (e.g. severe aortic stenosis)
Hypertrophic obstructive cardiomyopathy	Left ventricular hypertrophy, asymmetric septal hypertrophy, systolic anterior motion of the mitral valve, left ventricular outflow tract obstruction
Arrhythmogenic right ventricular dysplasia	Right ventricular dilatation, dysplasia

*Includes any cause of significant left ventricular dysfunction.

Systemic embolism

Differential diagnosis	Echo findings
Left atrial thrombus	Left atrial thrombus* or predisposing condition (e.g. mitral stenosis)
Mural thrombus	Left ventricular thrombus (usually regional akinesia)
Paradoxical embolus	Patent foramen ovale ± interatrial septum aneurysm
Atrial myxoma	Atrial myxoma
Endocarditis	Vegetation
Papillary fibroelastoma	Valvular mass
Prosthetic valve thrombus	Prosthesis dysfunction ± thrombus*
Aortic atheroma	Aortic atheroma >4 mm*

*Best seen on transoesophageal echocardiography.

Blunt trauma

Possible injuries	Echo findings
Myocardial contusion	Left ventricular dysfunction, regional wall motion abnormality, pericardial effusion
Coronary damage	Left ventricular dysfunction, regional wall motion abnormality
Myocardial rupture	Pericardial effusion/tamponade
Aortic dissection/rupture*	Dissection flap, aortic aneurysm, atrial regurgitation, pericardial effusion
Valvular dysfunction*	Leaflet tear, chordal or papillary rupture

*Best seen on transoesophageal echocardiography.

Reporting an echo study

After completing an echo study you should review all the images, perform necessary measurements/calculations, and review previous echoes if these are available. It is then possible to formulate a report.

An approach to reporting has already been covered for many important conditions, and this should be tailored to the findings of each patient. If all aspects of a study are completely normal, each structure should still be reported individually, including the minimal quantitative dataset, but detailed qualitative descriptions are not required. If significant pathology is present, the report should be as detailed as possible.

A comprehensive summary of the descriptive terms, measurements and analysis that should be included in a standard report has been issued by the American Society of Echocardiography (http://www.asefiles.org/Standardized_Echo_Report_Rev1.pdf).

The following information should form the basis of the report:

1. Patient information
    -   Patient name
    -   Date of birth
    -   Sex
    -   Unique identifier
    -   Height and weight: used to calculate body surface area
    -   Heart rate and rhythm (e.g. atrial fibrillation, left bundle branch block)
    -   Blood pressure
2. Quality statement
    -   Comment on quality of echo study
    -   Comment on views/data not obtained

3. Qualitative descriptions
   Comment on the structure, function and other relevant information about:
   - Left ventricle
   - Right ventricle
   - Atria and interatrial septum
   - Aortic valve
   - Mitral valve
   - Tricuspid valve
   - Pulmonary valve
   - Aorta
   - Pulmonary artery
   - Inferior vena cava
   - Pericardium
4. Quantitative data
   - Standard measurements and calculations, indexed to body surface area where possible
5. Summary of findings
   - Important positive and negative findings. 'Normal study' is acceptable if appropriate
6. Person performing and reporting echo

Normal values

The ranges of values for normal and abnormal are derived from the recommendations of the American Society of Echocardiography (2005). Normal values have been established for most echocardiographic parameters, and are most reliable when adjusted for body size.

Although different measures of body size have been proposed, the current recommendation is to use body surface area (BSA). This is derived from body mass and height as follows:

Body surface area (m^2) = $\sqrt{\text{height (cm)} \times \text{weight (kg)}/3600}$

Left ventricular dimensions

	Women				Men			
	Normal	Mild	Moderate	Severe	Normal	Mild	Moderate	Severe
LVIDd (cm)	3.9–5.3	5.4–5.7	5.8–6.1	≥6.2	4.2–5.9	6.0–6.3	6.4–6.8	≥6.9
LVIDd/BSA cm/m²	2.4–3.2	3.3–3.4	3.5–3.7	≥3.8	2.2–3.1	3.2–3.4	3.5–3.6	≥3.7
LVd volume (ml)	56–104	105–117	118–130	≥131	67–155	156–178	179–201	≥201
LVd volume/BSA (ml/m²)	35–75	76–86	87–96	≥97	35–75	76–86	87–96	≥97
LVs volume (ml)	19–49	50–59	60–69	≥70	22–58	59–70	71–82	≥83
LVs volume/BSA (ml/m²)	12–30	31–36	37–42	≥43	12–30	31–36	37–42	≥43
SWTd (cm)	0.6–0.9	1.0–1.2	1.3–1.5	≥1.6	0.6–1.0	1.1–1.3	1.4–1.6	≥1.7
PWTd (cm)	0.6–0.9	1.0–1.2	1.3–1.5	≥1.6	0.6–1.0	1.1–1.3	1.4–1.6	≥1.7
LVOT (cm)	1.8–2.4				1.8–2.4			

Left ventricular (LV) mass

Cubed method

	Women				Men			
LV mass (g)	67–162	163–186	187–210	≥211	88–224	225–258	259–292	≥293
LV mass/BSA (g/m²)	43–95	96–108	109–121	≥122	49–115	116–131	132–148	≥149

Area length method

	Women				Men			
LV mass (g)	66–150	151–171	172–182	≥183	96–200	201–227	228–254	≥255
LV mass/BSA (g/m²)	44–88	89–100	101–112	≥113	50–102	103–116	117–130	≥131

Left ventricular function

	Women				Men			
Fractional shortening (%)	27–45	22–26	17–21	≤16	25–43	20–24	15–19	≤14
Ejection fraction (%)	≥55	45–54	30–44	<30	≥55	45–54	30–44	<30

LVIDd, diastolic left ventricular internal diameter; BSA, body surface area; LV, left ventricle; d, diastolic; s, systolic; SWTd, PWT, posterior wall thickness; LVOT, left ventricular outflow tract.

Right ventricular (RV) dimensions

	Women				Men			
	Normal	Mild	Moderate	Severe	Normal	Mild	Moderate	Severe
RV basal diameter (cm)	2.0–2.8	2.9–3.3	3.4–3.8	≥3.9	2.0–2.8	2.9–3.3	3.4–3.8	≥3.9
Mid RV diameter (cm)	2.7–3.3	3.4–3.4	3.8–4.1	≥4.2	2.7–3.3	3.4–3.4	3.8–4.1	≥4.2
Base–apex (cm)	7.1–7.9	8.0–8.5	8.6–9.1	≥9.2	7.1–7.9	8.0–8.5	8.6–9.1	≥9.2
Right ventricular outflow tract diameter								
Subpulmonic (cm)	1.7–2.3	2.4–2.7	2.8–3.1	≥3.0	1.7–2.3	2.4–2.7	2.8–3.1	≥3.0
Supra-aortic (cm)	2.5–2.9	3.0–3.2	3.3–3.5	≥3.6	2.5–2.9	3.0–3.2	3.3–3.5	≥3.6
Pulmonary artery diameter (cm)	1.5–2.1	2.2–2.5	2.6–2.9	≥3.0	1.5–2.1	2.2–2.5	2.6–2.9	≥3.0
Right ventricular diastolic area (cm²)	11–28	29–32	33–37	≥38	11–28	29–32	33–37	≥38
Right ventricular systolic area (cm²)	7.5–16	17–19	20–22	≥23	7.5–16	17–19	20–22	≥23
Fractional area change (%)	32–60	25–31	18–24	≤17	32–60	25–31	18–24	≤17
Atrial dimensions								
LA diameter in PSLAX (cm)	2.7–3.8	3.9–4.2	4.3–4.6	≥4.7	3.0–4.0	4.1–4.6	4.7–5.2	≥5.2
LA diameter/BSA (cm/m²)	1.5–2.3	2.4–2.6	2.7–2.9	≥3.0	1.5–2.3	2.4–2.6	2.7–2.9	≥3.0
LA volume (ml)	22–52	53–62	63–72	≥73	18–58	59–68	69–78	≥79
LA area (cm²)	≤20	20–30	31–40	>40	≤20	20–30	31–40	>40
LA volume/BSA (ml/m²)	16–28	29–33	34–39	≥40	16–28	29–33	34–39	≥40
RA diameter (cm)	2.9–4.5	4.6–4.9	5.0–5.4	≥5.5	2.9–4.5	4.6–4.9	5.0–5.4	≥5.5
RA diameter/BSA (cm/m²)	1.7–2.5	2.6–2.8	2.9–3.1	≥3.2	1.7–2.5	2.6–2.8	2.9–3.1	≥3.2

LA, left atrium; PSLAX, parasternal long axis; BSA, body surface area; RA, right atrium.

Valve dimensions

	Normal	Mild	Moderate	Severe
Aortic annulus (cm)	2.3–2.9			
Mitral annulus (cm)	2.0–3.8			
Pulmonary annulus (cm)	1.8–2.2			
Tricuspid annulus (cm)	1.3–2.8			
Aortic valve area (cm^2)	3.0–4.0	2.5–1.5	1.5–1.0	< 1.0
Mitral valve area (cm^2)	4.0–6.0	2.0–1.6	1.5–1.0	< 1.0
Pulmonary valve area (cm^2)	3.0–5.0	2.0–1.0	0.5–1.0	< 0.5
Tricuspid valve area (cm^2)	4.0–6.0	2.0–1.6	1.5–1.1	≤ 1.0

Aortic dimensions

Sinus of Valsalva (cm)*	3.1–3.7
Ascending aorta (cm)	< 3.7
Ascending aorta (cm/m^2)	1.4–2.1
Descending aorta (cm/m^2)	1.0–1.6

*The normal range for aortic root can be estimated according to the following formulae:
< 19 years:
Aortic root diameter = 1.02 + (0.98 × BSA) (range ± 0.18)
20–39 years:
Aortic root diameter = 0.97 + (1.12 × BSA) (range ± 0.24)
≥ 40 years:
Aortic root diameter = 1.92 + (0.74 × BSA) (range ± 0.40)
(From Roman MJ, Devereux RB, Kramer-Fox R et al. American Journal of Cardiology 1989; 64: 507–512.)

Normal Doppler values

	Normal	Mild	Moderate	Severe
Aortic valve peak velocity (m/s)	≤ 2.5	2.6–2.9	3.0–4.0	> 4.0
Pulmonary valve peak velocity (m/s)	0.6–0.9	1.0–3.0	3.0–4.0	> 4.0
LVOT peak velocity (m/s)	0.7–1.1			
RVOT peak velocity (m/s)	0.6–0.9			

LVOT, left ventricular outflow tract; RVOT, right ventricular outflow tract.

Normal		
Mitral valve	< 50 years	> 50 years
E wave peak velocity (cm/s)	72 ± 14	62 ± 14
A wave peak velocity (cm/s)	40 ± 10	59 ± 14
E : A ratio	1.9 ± 0.6	1.1 ± 0.3
Deceleration time (ms)	179 ± 20	210 ± 36

Values are mean ± SD.

Normal		
Tricuspid valve	< 50 years	> 50 years
E wave peak velocity (cm/s)	51 ± 17	46 ± 13
A wave peak velocity (cm/s)	27 ± 8	33 ± 8
E : A ratio	2.0 ± 0.5	1.3 ± 0.4
Deceleration time (ms)	188 ± 22	198 ± 23

Values are mean ± SD.

Useful formulae

Basic physics

Properties of ultrasound

$$v = f\lambda$$

where v is the velocity of ultrasound wave, f is the ultrasound frequency and λ is the ultrasound wavelength.

Doppler formula

$$\Delta f = \frac{2f_0 v \cos\theta}{c}$$

where Δf is the Doppler frequency shift, f_0 is the ultrasound frequency from the transducer, θ is the angle between the ultrasound beam and blood flow, v is the velocity of blood flow and c is the velocity of ultrasound in tissue (1540 m/s).

Nyquist limit

$$\text{Nyquist limit (frequency)} = \frac{\text{pulse repetition frequency}}{2}$$

Left ventricular function

Fractional shortening

$$\text{Fractional shortening (\%)} = \frac{\text{LVIDd} - \text{LVIDs} \times 100}{\text{LVIDd}}$$

where LVIDd is the end diastolic left ventricular internal diameter and LVIDs is the end systolic diameter.

Ejection fraction

$$\text{Ejection fraction (\%)} = \frac{\text{stroke volume}}{\text{end diastolic volume}} \times 100$$

$$= \frac{\text{end diastolic volume} - \text{end systolic volume}}{\text{end diastolic volume}} \times 100$$

Simpson's biplane formula

$$\text{Left ventricular volume (ml)} = \sum [\pi(ai \times bi)L/4n]$$

where ai and bi are the diameters of the cylinder from two orthogonal views (cm), L/n is the height of the disc (cm) and n is the number of discs.

Left ventricular hypertrophy

Cubed formula

$$\text{Left ventricular mass (g)} = 0.80 \times [1.04 \times (\text{IVSd} + \text{PWTd} + \text{LVIDd})^3 - (\text{LVIDd})^3] + 0.6 \text{ g}$$

where the specific gravity of muscle is 1.04 g/cm^3, IVSd is the end diastolic inter-ventricular septal thickness, LVIDd is the end diastolic left ventricular internal diameter and PWTd is the end diastolic posterior wall thickness.

Area–length formula

$$\text{Left ventricular mass (g)} = 1.05[(5/6)A_1(L+T)(5/6)A_2L]$$

where 1.05 g/ml is the specific gravity of muscle, A_1 and A_2 are the epicardial and endocardial parasternal short axis areas (cm^2), respectively, L is the length from the apex to the mid-point of the mitral annulus (cm) and T is the average wall thickness calculated from A_1 and A_2 (cm).

Truncated ellipsoid

Left ventricular mass (g)

$$= 1.05[(b+T)^2\{2/3(a+T)+d-d^3/[3(a+T)^2]\} - b^2(2/3a+dd^3/3a^2)]$$

where 1.05 g/ml is the specific gravity of muscle, b is the minor axis radius of the left ventricle measured at the level of the papillary muscle tip (cm), a is the major axis from the apex to the intersection of the maximal minor axis (cm) and d is the major axis from this intersection to the mid-point of the mitral annular plane (cm). T is the average wall thickness derived from the epicardial and endocardial short axis areas, A_1 and A_2 (cm).

Quantitative Doppler echocardiography

Stroke volume (SV)

$$\text{Left ventricular SV (ml)} = \text{VTI}_{\text{LVOT}} \times \pi r_{\text{LVOT}}^2$$

where VTI_{LVOT} is the velocity time integral of forward flow at the left ventricular outflow tract (cm/s), and r_{LVOT} is the radius of the left ventricular outflow tract (cm).

$$\text{Right ventricular SV (ml)} = \text{VTI}_{\text{RVOT}} \times \pi r_{\text{RVOT}}^2$$

where VTI_{RVOT} is the velocity time integral of forward flow at the right ventricular outflow tract (cm/s), and r_{RVOT} is the radius of the right ventricular outflow tract (cm).

Cardiac output

$$\text{Cardiac output (ml/min)} = \text{left ventricular SV} \times \text{heart rate}$$

Regurgitant volume

$$\text{Regurgitant volume (ml)} = \text{total forward flow} - \text{SV}$$

Regurgitant fraction

$$\text{Regurgitant fraction (\%)} = \frac{\text{total forward flow} - \text{SV} \times 100}{\text{total forward flow}}$$

Shunt ratio

$$\text{Shunt ratio} = \frac{\text{right ventricular SV}}{\text{left ventricular SV}}$$

Valvular disease

Continuity equation

$$\text{Area}_{\text{AV}} (\text{cm}^2) = \frac{(\pi \, \text{radius}_{\text{LVOT}}^2) \times \text{VTI}_{\text{LVOT}}}{\text{VTI}_{\text{AV}}}$$

where area_{AV} is the aortic valve area, $\text{radius}_{\text{LVOT}}$ is the radius of the left ventricular outflow tract (cm), and VTI_{AV} and VTI_{LVOT} are the velocity time integrals of the aortic valve and left ventricular outflow tract, respectively (cm/s).

Proximal isovelocity surface area (PISA)

$$\text{EROA (cm}^2) = \frac{(2\pi r^2) \times V_a}{V_{max}}$$

where EROA is effective regurgitant orifice area, r is the radius of the proximal isovelocity surface area, V_a is the aliasing velocity and V_{max} is the peak velocity of regurgitant flow.

PISA lite (mitral regurgitation only)

$$\text{EROA} = r^2/2$$

where EROA is effective regurgitant orifice area, r is the radius of the proximal isovelocity surface area, with the aliasing velocity set at 40 cm/s.

Regurgitant volume

$$\text{Regurgitant volume} = \text{EROA} \times \text{VTI}_{max}$$

where EROA is effective regurgitant orifice area and VTI_{max} is the velocity time integral of the maximal regurgitant flow.

Index

Page numbers followed by 'f' indicate figures, 't' indicate tables, and 'b' indicate boxes.